QBASE PAEDIATRICS: 1

MCQs FOR THE MRCPCH

QBASE PAEDIATRICS: 1

MCQs FOR THE MRCPCH

Rachel U. Sidwell MRCP MRCPCH DFFP DA
London, UK

Mike Thomson MRCP FRCPCH DCH MD
London, UK

With a contribution by
Kamal Patel

QBase series developed and edited by

Edward J. Hammond MA BM BCh MRCP FRCA
Shackleton Department of Anaesthetics
Southampton University Hospital NHS Trust

Andrew K. McIndoe MC ChB FRCA
Sir Humphry Davy Department of Anaesthesia
Bristol Royal Infirmary

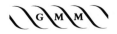

© 2001
Greenwich Medical Media Ltd.
137 Euston Road
London
NW1 2AA

ISBN 1 84110 044 7

First Published 2001

A catalogue record for this book is available from the British Library

Produced and Designed by
Saxon Graphics Limited, Derby

Printed in Great Britain by
Ashford Colour Press Ltd, Hants

CONTENTS

Preface

The MRCPCH Part I examination is composed of 60 multiple choice stem questions each with 5 parts (in reality, 300 individual questions in total), designed to test a candidates breadth of knowledge. The key to passing multiple choice question (MCQ) examinations is to practice doing as many MCQs as possible. This book makes practising a little more fun via its free interactive CD-ROM. The book is composed of 5 practice exams, each of 60 five-part MCQs, covering the range of paediatric sub-specialities and providing examples of the types of question encountered in the MRCPCH. All of the questions in the book are also included on the CD-ROM.

The CD-ROM enables the questions to be scrambled randomly to create new exams, and prevent memorisation purely from page position. Also, for methodical learning, questions on a particular subject can be selected separately, and a pure topic covered in detail. This way, we hope you will feel you are getting somewhere!

Read each question carefully; do not be caught out by simple phraseology, as this is extremely annoying, and examiners seem to enjoy it. Look for key phrases, such as 'always' (extremely unlikely to be correct) and 'never' (also very unlikely). Some terms such as 'commonly', 'usually', and 'often' are unfortunately ambiguous and open to varied interpretation. Beware of double negatives.

Interestingly the exam is now positively marked. This means the agony of deciding whether or not to answer a question is removed. All questions should now be answered, even when you have absolutely no idea of the answer, as points will not be deducted for an incorrect one. Remember that even when you are very unsure of an answer, your probability of being right is more than that of being wrong, simply because you are giving an educated guess. But always guess *intelligently*.

Wishing you the best of luck,

Rachel Sidwell
Mike Thomson

London, March 2001

Editor's note

The MRCPCH Part I examination is now **non-negatively marked**, correct answers scoring 1 point and incorrect answers 0 points (as opposed to -1 points in the previous negatively-marked system). The version of the QBase Interactive Examination software used on the enclosed CD-ROM, called **QBasePlus**, marks your MCQ attempts and stores your scores in exactly the same way, to provide a realistic examination simulation.

Non-negative marking is designed to remove the penalty for making an incorrect answer, and encourage a response to every question. As the authors remark in their preface, with knowledge and practice of MCQs, you can skew the probability of being right in your favour, by *guessing intelligently*.

Good luck!

Edward Hammond
Andrew McIndoe

QBase Series Developers/Editors
March 2001

RUNNING THE QBasePlus
PROGRAM ON CD-ROM

SYSTEM REQUIREMENTS

An IBM compatible PC with a minimum 80386 processor and 4MB of RAM VGA Monitor set up to display at least 256 colours.

CD-ROM drive

Windows 3.1 or higher with Microsoft compatible mouse

The display setting of your computer must be set to display "SMALL FONTS".

See Windows manuals for further instructions on how to do this.

INSTALLATION INSTRUCTIONS

The program will install the appropriate files onto your hard drive. It requires the QBasePlus CD-ROM to be installed in the D:\drive.

In order to run QBasePlus the CD-ROM must be in the drive.

Print Readme.txt and Helpfile.txt on the CD-ROM for fuller instructions and user manual

Windows 95/98/2000

1. Insert the QBase CD-ROM into drive D:

2. From the **Start Menu**, select the **RUN** option

3. Type **D:\setup.exe** and press enter or return

4. Follow the instructions given by the installation program. Select the **Typical** Installation Option and accept the default directory for installation of QBasePlus. The installation program creates a folder called **QBasePlus** containing the program icon and another called **Exams** into which you can save previous exam attempts.

5. To run QBasePlus double click the **QBasePlus** icon in the QBasePlus folder. From Windows Explorer double click the **QBasePlus.exe** file in the QBasePlus folder or go to Windows Start menu, Programs, QBasePlus then **QBasePlus.exe**

Windows 3.1/Windows for Workgroups 3.11

1. Insert the QBase CD-ROM into drive D:

2. From the **File Menu**, select the **RUN** option

3. Type **D:\setup.exe** and press enter or return

4. Follow the instruction given by the installation program. Select the **Typical** Installation Option and accept the default directory for installation of QBasePlus. The installation program creates a program window and directory called **QBasePlus** containing the program icon. It also creates a directory called **Exams** into which you can save previous exam attempts.

5. To run QBasePlus double click the **QBasePlus** icon in the QBasePlus program manager window. From File Manager double click the **QBasePlus.exe** file in the QBasePlus directory.

Exam 1: Questions

QUESTION 1

Reversed splitting of the second heart sound is heard in

- **A.** Atrial septal defect
- **B.** Pulmonary hypertension
- **C.** Tetralogy of Fallot
- **D.** Aortic stenosis
- **E.** Left bundle branch block

QUESTION 2

The following are true regarding a patent ductus arteriosus

- **A.** The ECG may be indistinguishable from that of a VSD
- **B.** The chest X-ray may be normal
- **C.** Maternal Warfarin therapy is associated
- **D.** It should be closed even if asymptomatic
- **E.** A collapsing pulse is present

QUESTION 3

Jervell–Lang–Nielson syndrome

- **A.** Is an autosomal dominant condition
- **B.** Is associated with myopia
- **C.** Repeat drop attacks occur
- **D.** Has a better prognosis than Romano-Ward syndrome
- **E.** β-blockers reduce the mortality significantly

QUESTION 4

Left isomerism

- **A.** Involves asplenia
- **B.** Is usually more severe than right isomerism
- **C.** Is usually associated with severe congenital heart disease
- **D.** Involves two right lungs
- **E.** Is associated with maternal Warfarin therapy

QUESTION 5

The following will cause a decreased transfer factor for carbon monoxide

A. Anaemia
B. Polycythaemia
C. Pneumonia
D. Pulmonary fibrosis
E. Exercise

QUESTION 6

Pulmonary tuberculosis

A. Is usually symptomatic in children
B. Is visible as calcification of the primary focus on chest X-ray 2 months after infection
C. Is more likely to become disseminated in young children
D. Is usually best investigated in children with gastric aspirates
E. Is highly infectious in children

QUESTION 7

Regarding pulse oximetry

A. Hyperbilirubinaemia does not affect SpO_2
B. It can be used for assessment of collateral circulation prior to arterial cannulation
C. Green and blue nail varnish result in lower SpO_2 readings
D. A left shift in the oxyhaemoglobin dissociation curve will give a falsely low SpO_2 reading
E. High levels of methaemoglobin always result in erroneously low SpO_2 readings

QUESTION 8

The following are true about gastric acid production

A. Sympathomimetics increase gastric acid production
B. Secretin inhibits gastic acid production
C. *Helicobacter pylori* colonisation of the gastric lining increases gastric acid production
D. Vagal nerve stimulation increases the pH of the intragastric milieu
E. Pancreatic β-cells increase the pH of the intragastric milieu

QUESTION 9

In an infant with intestinal lymphangiectasia

A. A small bowel biopsy will reveal minimal or no lacteals
B. The cause may be constrictive pericarditis
C. An association is Klippel-Trenauney-Weber syndrome
D. Faecal α-1 anti-trypsin may be decreased
E. Mental retardation and regression are common

QUESTION 10

Chronic pancreatitis in children

A. Occurs in ascariasis
B. Occurs in Wilson's disease
C. Will display Cullen's sign if prolonged
D. Is predisposed to by cystinosis
E. Is predisposed to by cystinuria

QUESTION 11

The following are true of children with chronic constipation

A. Anal sphincter tone is increased
B. Diarrhoea is suggestive of an underlying aetiology such as coeliac disease
C. There is a male preponderance
D. Increased fat intake will increase gut velocity and aid in management
E. There is an association with cow's milk intolerance/allergy

QUESTION 12

When a urinary tract abnormality in a foetus is diagnosed by antenatal ultrasound

A. No action is required if the ultrasound at 2 weeks postnatal age is normal
B. Bilateral hydronephrosis in a boy is most commonly due to Prune Belly syndrome
C. Unilateral hydronephrosis may require urgent surgery
D. Obstruction at the pelvi-ureteric junction requires foetal surgery even if the kidney is functioning well
E. Autosomal recessive polycystic kidney disease may cause a Potter's phenotype

QUESTION 13

Urinary tract infections

A. Occur in 5% of boys and 9% of girls
B. Have a predisposing structural renal lesion in 20%
C. Occurring for the first time in an 8 month old usually signify a structural abnormality
D. Require pyuria to establish the diagnosis
E. Do not require investigation until there is a recurrence

QUESTION 14

Alport's syndrome

A. May be effectively treated by plasmapheresis
B. Is diagnosed by electronmicroscopy of a renal biopsy
C. May cause retinal defects similar to congenital toxoplasmosis
D. Is the result of spontaneous mutation in 20% of cases
E. Involves high frequency deafness which progresses to the whole speech range

QUESTION   15

In a child with chronic renal failure

A. Salt-wasting is common
B. Eggs and milk are acceptable safe sources of protein
C. Somatic growth is maintained until glomerular filtration rate falls below 20% of normal
D. Nutritional supplementation of both water- and fat-soluble vitamins is necessary
E. Osteodystrophy is associated with high phosphate levels and secondary hyperparathyroidism

QUESTION   16

Recognised poor prognostic factors in children presenting with fulminant liver failure include

A. Age under 10 years
B. Paracetamol-induced liver failure
C. Marked hepatomegaly with evidence of portal hypertension
D. Urine output of less than 0.3 ml/kg/hour
E. Parents who are consanguinous

QUESTION   17

In a child or adolescent diagnosed with Wilson's disease which of the following are true

A. Acute psychosis may be the only presenting feature
B. 24 hour copper excretion is markedly reduced after administration of penicillamine
C. All first degree family members should be screened for pre-symptomatic disease
D. There is a 72% chance of association with HLA A3
E. Penicillamine is the treatment of choice

QUESTION   18

Treatment of potential or actual variceal bleeding in childhood can involve the following

A. Transjugular intrahepatic porto-systemic shunt
B. Endoscopic variceal band ligation
C. With a Sengstaken-Blakemore tube, use of the oesophageal balloon only
D. Neomycin for gut sterilisation to aid in the prevention of hepatic encephalopathy
E. Intravenous octreotide infusion

QUESTION   19

In conjugated hyperbilirubinaemia in infancy

A. Choledochal cysts are the second commonest surgical cause
B. Due to biliary atresia, a rapid rise in urobilinogen is seen on the first day
C. Due to tyrosinaemia, urinary succinylacetone is a reliable diagnostic tool
D. Due to α-1 anti-trypsin deficiency, liver involvement is commonly accompanied by intra-uterine growth retardation
E. Kasai portoenterostomy is not effective for intrahepatic biliary atresia even if performed before 60 days of age

QUESTION 20

Haemorrhagic disease of the newborn

A. Is due to low Vitamin C-dependant clotting factors
B. Always presents during the first week of life
C. Is not associated with fatal haemorrhage
D. Is particularly seen in babies fed on bottled milk
E. Is more common if the mother is on a liver enzyme inducing drug

QUESTION 21

In glucose-6-phosphate dehydrogenase (G6PD) deficiency

A. G6PD levels may be normal during a crisis
B. Females may be clinically affected
C. Type A (African type) is the more severe form
D. G6PD is an enzyme involved in the Emden-Meyerhof pathway
E. Bite cells are seen during a crisis

QUESTION 22

In Beta-thalassaemia major

A. Excess β chains precipitate
B. Fetal haemoglobin is increased
C. Golf-ball cells are seen on the blood film
D. Bone marrow transplant may be indicated
E. A "hair on end" skull X-ray appearance is seen

QUESTION 23

In Haemophilia A

A. Prophylactic recombinant factor VIII therapy is used
B. The prothrombin time is prolonged
C. 50% of patients have no family history
D. Factor VIII antibodies occur in around 10% of haemophiliacs
E. Carrier females usually have normal factor VIII levels

QUESTION 24

The following are true of vincristine

A. It is a folic acid antagonist
B. It may cause SIADH
C. Its effects can be reversed with vitamin B_6
D. It may cause lung fibrosis
E. It may cause a peripheral neuropathy

QUESTION 25

In retinoblastoma

A. The hereditary form is associated with deletions of chromosome 13p
B. All hereditary tumours are bilateral
C. Unilateral tumours are usually diagnosed earlier than bilateral tumours
D. Management may be with radiotherapy
E. The hereditary form is associated with soft tissue sarcomas

QUESTION 26

IgE

A. Has two distinct subclasses
B. Is involved in type I hypersensitivity reactions
C. Is present in the circulation as a pentamer
D. Is raised in Duncan's syndrome
E. A serum level of 10 000 IU/ml is diagnostic for the hyper IgE syndrome

QUESTION 27

The DiGeorge anomaly

A. May involve oesophageal atresia
B. Usually presents with infections
C. Involves predominantly a decrease in the number and function of T cells
D. Results from a failure of development of the 2nd branchial arch
E. Involves a microdeletion of chromosome 20q11

QUESTION 28

Chronic granulomatous disease

A. Is an autosomal recessive condition
B. Is due to a failure of superoxide production
C. Is associated with granulomas in the liver
D. Is associated with gingival hyperplasia
E. The main immune defect is of T cell origin

QUESTION 29

The following vaccines are live attenuated

A. Measles
B. Pertussis
C. BCG
D. Yellow fever
E. Influenza

QUESTION   30

In the toxic shock syndrome (TSS)

A. Creatinine kinase levels are raised
B. It is due to toxins produced by *Staphylococcus aureus* phage group II
C. The diagnostic criteria include toxic actions in 3 or more systems
D. Diarrhoea is rarely present
E. Group A streptococcus may cause a similar clinical picture

QUESTION   31

Enterobius vermiculata

A. Causes ileo-caecal obstruction
B. Is a whipworm
C. Is diagnosed by the Sellotape test
D. Is a cause of pruritus ani
E. Is treated with piperazine

QUESTION   32

Regarding varicella-zoster infection

A. The incidence of varicella is seasonal with a peak from March to May
B. The infectious period may be prolonged in immunocompromised individuals
C. Shingles (zoster) is caused by reactivation of the patient's own varicella virus, and is transmissable to others as chicken pox
D. Even after VZIG prophylaxis, about half of neonates exposed will become infected
E. Up to 40% of under 16 years old with no history of chicken pox are varicella-zoster antibody positive

QUESTION   33

Regarding phenylketonuria

A. It has an incidence of 1 in 1000
B. It involves a block in the metabolic pathway converting tyrosine to dopamine
C. Blood phenylalanine levels are raised from birth
D. The appearance of fair hair and skin, and blue eyes, is always seen
E. A low phenylalanine diet must be adhered to until teenage years

QUESTION   34

Pompe disease

A. Is a glycogen storage disease
B. Involves severe hypoglycaemia as a feature
C. Involves cardiomyopathy as a feature
D. Is diagnosed by plasma amino acid profile
E. Includes a late onset form with myopathy

QUESTION   35

Hepatorenal tyrosinaemia

A. Has an acute and a chronic form
B. Is more commonly seen in Morrocans
C. Includes renal Fanconi syndrome and hepatocellular degeneration
D. May be treated with NTBC
E. A raised α-FP is seen

QUESTION   36

During normal puberty in boys

A. Onset is normally from 8–11 years
B. The first sign is pubic hair development
C. The growth spurt occurs at around 11.5 years
D. Early development of secondary sexual characteristics in boys is usually familial
E. A testicular volume of 4 ml indicates the onset of puberty

QUESTION   37

The following are features of neonatal hyperthyroidism

A. Macroglossia
B. Infant large for gestational age
C. Neonatal jaundice
D. Microcephaly
E. Postmaturity

QUESTION   38

The following may result in hyponatraemia

A. Carbamazepine
B. Glibenclamide
C. Cystic fibrosis
D. Ewing's sarcoma
E. Cyclophosphamide

QUESTION 39

In congenital adrenal hyperplasia due to 21-hydroxylase deficiency, there are raised plasma levels of

A. Sodium
B. Aldosterone
C. Cortisol
D. Androstenedione
E. Testosterone

QUESTION 40

The facial nerve

A. Passes through the stylomastoid foramen
B. Conveys secretomotor fibres to the sublingual salivary glands
C. Has a motor nucleus located in the medulla
D. Transmits taste fibres from the posterior two thirds of the tongue
E. A unilateral lesion of the motor nucleus affects the lower part of the ipsilateral face only

QUESTION 41

The following are signs which are of concern regarding development

A. No words at 18 months
B. Echolalia at 2 years of age
C. Demonstration of hand dominance in a child under 1 year
D. Absent pincer grasp at 18 months
E. Bottom shuffling at 18 months

QUESTION 42

Lennox-Gastaut syndrome

A. Usually has an onset under 3 years of age
B. Is a syndrome of loss of language skills associated with seizures
C. Has EEG findings of slow spike and wave forms
D. Constitutes a large proportion of the children with intractable epilepsy
E. Involves normal development until the onset of seizures

QUESTION 43

In myotonic dystrophy

A. The heart is not affected
B. Mental retardation is uncommon
C. Frontal baldness is seen in males
D. Cataracts are a feature
E. Children born to carrier fathers are more severely affected

QUESTION 44

The following may present as an acute abdomen

A. Lead poisoning
B. Henoch-Schönlein purpura
C. Sickle cell disease
D. Pneumonia
E. Congenital spherocytosis

QUESTION 45

Vigabatrin

A. Enhances gabergic activity in the brain
B. Has antidepressant effects
C. Suppresses EEG abnormality and seizures in infantile spasms
D. Exacerbates seizures of localised onset
E. May cause ocular cataract

QUESTION 46

Frusemide

A. Has a rapid onset but long-lasting action
B. Is of proven benefit in treating chronic lung disease of the newborn
C. May cause hyperkalaemia
D. May cause renal calculi with long-term use in neonates
E. Can be used to manage hypercalcaemia

QUESTION 47

The following are true regarding macrolide antibiotics

A. Erythromycin is bacteriostatic
B. They are the first choice of treatment in community-acquired atypical pneumonia
C. Erythromycin may cause intestinal ileus
D. They may cause cholestatic hepatitis
E. They can be administered with terfinadine but not with astemizole

QUESTION 48

The following are true regarding drug metabolism inhibition

A. Allopurinol inhibits azathioprine metabolism
B. Sodium valproate inhibits lamotrigine metabolism
C. Griseofulvin inhibits propanolol metabolism
D. Isoniazid inhibits pyridoxine metabolism
E. Amoxycillin inhibits warfarin metabolism

QUESTION 49

Erythema multiforme

A. Is commonly triggered by herpes simplex virus infection
B. Classically presents with target lesions
C. Has a severe form known as Stevens-Johnson syndrome
D. May become bullous
E. May be caused by leukaemia

QUESTION 50

Regarding autoantibodies

A. Rheumatoid factor is an antibody to the Fab portion of IgG
B. Anti-centromere antibody is seen in CREST syndrome
C. Anti-histone antibody is seen particulary in drug-induced lupus
D. p-ANCA is specific to Wegener's granulomatosis
E. RhF may be positive in endocarditis

QUESTION 51

Subcutaneous nodules are found in

A. Churg-Strauss syndrome
B. Reiter's syndrome
C. RhF positive polyarticular JCA
D. Rheumatic fever
E. Juvenile ankylosing spondylitis

QUESTION 52

Regarding Amyloidosis

A. Familial Mediterranean fever is associated with amyloidosis
B. In secondary amyloidosis, the amyloid is homologous with immunoglobulin κ or λ chains
C. Tissue biopsy is stained with Congo red dye and is orange under polarising light
D. Secondary amyloidosis is associated with systemic JCA
E. Nephrotic syndrome may be seen in secondary amyloidosis

QUESTION 53

The following conditions are inherited in an autosomal recessive fashion

A. Klinefelter syndrome
B. Duchenne muscular dystrophy
C. Familial hypophosphataemic rickets
D. Marfan's syndrome
E. Homocystinuria

QUESTION 54

The following inherited conditions and congenital cardiac malformations are associated

A. CHARGE association - Hypertrophic cardiomyopathy
B. Neurofibromatosis – Peripheral pulmonary stenosis
C. Holt-Oram syndrome - Primum ASD
D. Chromosome 22 microdeletion - Truncus arteriosus
E. Hunter syndrome - Tetralogy of Fallot

QUESTION 55

In the embryological development of the cardiovascular system

A. Development is from endodermal origin
B. The ductus arteriosus forms from the remnant of the 6th right aortic arch
C. The heart chambers are formed by the end of the 6th week
D. The ascending limb of the cardiac loop gives rise to the left ventricle
E. The heart begins to beat at around 23 days

QUESTION 56

The following are correct in a Normal distribution

A. The mode and the mean are equal
B. The standard deviation is a measure of how accurately the calculated mean approaches the true population mean
C. The median is greater than the mean
D. 68% of values lie within +/- one standard deviation of the mean
E. The standard error of the mean is calculated by dividing the mean by the square root of the sample size

QUESTION 57

The following definitions are correct

A. Neonatal mortality rate is the number of deaths of infants within 28 days of birth per 1000 of all births
B. Infant mortality rate is the number of deaths between 28 days and 1 year per 1000 live births
C. Perinatal mortality rate is the number of stillbirths plus deaths within the first 6 days per 1000 births (live and still)
D. Stillbirth rate is the number of stillbirths per 1000 of all births (live and still)
E. A neonate is an infant below 38 days old

QUESTION 58

Umbilical hernia in infancy is associated with the following

A. Beckwith-Weidemann syndrome
B. Turner's syndrome
C. Hypothyroidism
D. Pierre-Robin sequence
E. Prematurity

QUESTION 59

Maternal serum α-fetoprotein is increased in the following conditions

A. Trisomy 18
B. Intrauterine growth retardation
C. Cystic hygroma
D. Epidermolysis bullosa
E. Multiple pregnancy

QUESTION 60

The following are true

A. The mean airway pressure is the average pressure to which the lungs are expanded during the respiratory cycle
B. An increase in the gas flow rate will cause a fall in the pCO_2
C. A high PEEP can impede carbon dioxide elimination
D. Increasing the peak inspiratory pressure (PIP) will cause a fall in the pCO_2
E. The pO_2 is the percentage of oxygen that is bound with haemoglobin

Exam 1: Answers

QUESTION 1

A. FALSE B. FALSE C. FALSE D. TRUE E. TRUE

A reversed (paradoxical) splitting of the second heart sound is heard in aortic stenosis, left bundle branch block and hypertrophic obstructive cardiomyopathy (HOCM).

A wide fixed splitting is heard in atrial septal defect.

Wide mobile splitting is heard in pulmonary hypertension.

In tetralogy of Fallot a single second heart sound is heard (there is a soft P2) with an ejection systolic murmur at the upper left sternal edge due to flow through the pulmonary valve.

QUESTION 2

A. TRUE B. TRUE C. TRUE D. TRUE E. TRUE

A patent ductus arteriosus (PDA) is associated with congenital rubella syndrome and maternal warfarin therapy. It is commoner in girls, and in sick premature infants. In preterm infants there is a systolic murmur at the left sternal edge, a collapsing pulse and heart failure may develop. The ECG is usually normal, and the CXR may be normal or features of cardiac failure may be present. Older children usually have a continuous (machinary) murmur.

All PDAs should be closed because of the risk of endocarditis.

Medical management may be successful in neonates (indomethacin and fluid restriction). Surgical ligation is necessary if medical management fails or is not appropriate.

QUESTION 3

A. FALSE B. FALSE C. TRUE D. FALSE E. TRUE

Jervell-Lang-Nielson syndrome is a congenital cause of the prolonged QT syndrome. It is inherited as autosomal recessive and involves a long QT with congenital deafness. Repeat drop attacks occur with the episodes of arrhythmias. These may be triggered by excitement, fear or exercise.

Romano-Ward syndrome is an autosomal dominant condition of isolated prolonged QT syndrome and has a better prognosis.

β-blockers reduce the mortality of congenital prolonged QT syndromes from around 80% to around 6%.

QUESTION 4

Right
asplenia

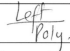
Left
Poly.

A. FALSE   B. FALSE   C. TRUE   D. FALSE   E. FALSE

Left isomerism is also known as polysplenia syndrome. Multiple small spleens are seen, bilateral left lungs, and there is no intrahepatic portion of the IVC.

Isomerism is usually associated with severe congenital heart disease. Right isomerism is usually more severe than left isomerism.

Right isomerism (aplsenia syndrome) involves no spleen, a central liver and two right lungs.

QUESTION 5

A. TRUE   B. FALSE   C. TRUE   D. TRUE   E. FALSE

The transfer factor for carbon monoxide (Dco) is a function of both the lung membrane diffusing capacity and pulmonary vascular components, which reflect the alveolar–capillary unit.

Diseases that compromise this will cause a decrease in the Dco. These include pulmonary vascular disease, anaemia, interstitial lung disease (e.g. pneumonia, pulmonary fibrosis) and obstructive airway disease.

Polycythaemia and exercise cause an increase in the transfer factor because of the increased amount of haemoglobin in the lung.

QUESTION 6

A. FALSE   B. FALSE   C. TRUE   D. TRUE   E. FALSE

Pulmonary tuberculosis is usually asymptomatic in children. The chest X-ray is normal in uncomplicated infection until the primary lung focus calcifies after 6 months to 1 year. Disseminated infection is more likely to occur in young children and in the immunocompromised.

Investigation to isolate TB in children is usually best obtained using gastric aspirates.

Pulmonary TB is not infectious in children though it is highly infectious in adults.

QUESTION 7

A. TRUE   B. TRUE   C. TRUE   D. FALSE   E. FALSE

Pulse oximetry is a non-invasive method of measuring the oxygen saturation of haemoglobin in pulsatile blood vessels, using both spectrophotometry and plethysmography (pulse volume), and can therefore be used to assess circulation. A photodetector is placed opposite a light emitting diode transmitting light at 660 nm (red) and 940 nm (infared). Saturation is measured by comparing the absorption of the two wavelengths by oxy- and deoxy-haemoglobin. Green and blue nail varnish increase the light absorbance at the 660nm wavelength, and thus result in lower readings.

A left shift in the oxyhaemoglobin dissociation curve results in a falsely *high* pO_2.

Methaemoglobin can result in either under or over estimation of the SpO_2, depending on whether the actual pO_2 is high or low.

QUESTION 8

A. FALSE   B. TRUE   C. FALSE   D. FALSE   E. FALSE

Helicobacter pylori can increase or decrease gastric acid, hence when it is eradicated in some individuals, acid production can actually increase compared to the preceding achlorhydria and the symptoms of gastro-oesophageal reflux will worsen. Insulin-secreting β-cells of the pancreas have no measurable effect on gastric acid production. It is increased by vagal stimulation, gastrin release, histamine release effecting H_2 receptors on oxyntic cells, and pepsin. It is decreased by low gastric pH, fear or sympathetic drive, and intestinal peptides such as cholecystokinin (pancreozymin), secretin, etc.

Ref: Murphy S, Aynsley-Green A, Wershil B Chapters 4 and 5. *Pediatric Gastrointestinal Disease*. Ed Walker et al. Mosby. St Louis 1996.

QUESTION 9

A. FALSE B. TRUE C. TRUE D. FALSE E. FALSE

Lacteals are dilated and villi are distorted on small bowel biopsy. Faecal α-1 anti-trypsin is a good marker of faecal protein loss and is therefore increased in intestinal lymphangiectasia. Learning difficulties and developmental regression occur in abetalipoproteinaemia.

QUESTION 10

A. TRUE B. TRUE C. FALSE D. TRUE E. TRUE

Cullen's sign is a bluish periumbilical area seen in acute haemorrhagic pancreatitis.

Ref: Gaskin K. Chapter 29. In: *Pediatric Gastrointestinal Disease*. Ed Walker et al. Mosby. St Louis. 1996.

QUESTION 11

A. FALSE B. FALSE C. FALSE D. FALSE E. TRUE

Anal sphincter tone is increased in Hirschsprung's disease. Overflow diarrhoea can occur with simple chronic constipation and does not indicate necessarily any other underlying pathology. Fat will slow GI transit and increased fluid and fibre should be recommended.

Ref: Murphy S, Claydon G. Chapter 20. In: *Pediatric Gastrointestinal Disease*. Ed Walker A et al. St Louis. 1996.

QUESTION 12

A. FALSE B. FALSE C. FALSE D. FALSE E. TRUE

Bilateral hydronephrosis in a boy is most likely to be due to posterior urethral valves. Unilateral hydronephrosis will require investigation and antibiotic prophylaxis but not urgent postnatal surgery. Similarly, in a well-functioning kidney no antenatal intervention is necessary.

QUESTION 13

A. FALSE B. FALSE C. TRUE D. FALSE E. FALSE

UTIs occur in most reported series at a frequency of 3% in girls and 1% in boys. A structural lesion is reported in 50% of cases. A pure growth of more than 100,000/ml signifies infection without white cells evident. Investigative regimens differ but all UTIs should be investigated with ultrasound initially.

QUESTION   14

A. FALSE   B. TRUE   C. FALSE   D. TRUE   E. TRUE

Do not get confused with the autoimmune disease Goodpasture's syndrome which has autoantibodies to lung and glomerular basement membrane, and is amenable to plasmapheresis treatment in certain cases. The typical electron-microscopic appearance is splitting of the basement membrane, so-called 'basket-weave' appearance. Eye defects include cataracts, anterior lenticonus, and macular lesions. X-linked dominant, autosomal dominant, or spontaneous mutation up to 20% may be the routes of inheritance.

QUESTION   15

A. TRUE   B. TRUE   C. FALSE   D. TRUE   E. TRUE

Egg and milk proteins have a high biological value and therefore uraemia from metabolism into nitrogenous waste is less. Growth rate is diminshed if GFR is less than 50% of normal. Poor diet due to anorexia or loss in dialysis may account for low water soluble vitamin levels, and vitamin D supplements may be required in the case of associated osteodystrophy. Renal osteodystrophy shows a high phosphate, low calcium, low alkaline phosphatase, and secondary hyperparathyroidism.

QUESTION   16

A. TRUE   B. TRUE   C. FALSE   D. TRUE   E. FALSE

Recognised poor prognostic factors are: age under 10 years; shrinking liver size and falling transaminase levels; concomitant renal failure; paracetamol-induced liver failure; onset of liver failure less than 7 days from initial presentation. Consanguinity allows autosomal recessive conditions to surface but liver failure resulting from conditions such as tyrosinaemia or organic acidaemias do not have a worse prognosis than other causes.

Ref: Alonso E, Superina R, Whitington P. Chapter 5. In: *Diseases of the liver and biliary system in childhood*. Ed Kelly D. Blackwell Science. Oxford 1999.

QUESTION   17

A. TRUE   B. FALSE   C. TRUE   D. FALSE   E. TRUE

After administration of penicillamine, the 24 hour urinary copper excretion, which is already raised, increases even more. Serum caeruloplasmin is raised and serum copper can be raised or normal. Liver biopsy characteristically reveals marked periportal copper deposition, and more recently the gene has been mapped to chromosome 13q 14-21. As it is autosomal dominant, other family members should be screened. The underlying mechanism appears to be a defect of hepatocyte transport of copper into the caeruloplasmin compartment. HLA-A3 is found in association with 72% of haemochromatosis – HLA-B7 in Australia and HLA-B14 in France are also seen.

Ref: Tanner S. Chapter 10. In: *Disorders of the liver and biliary system in childhood*. Ed Kelly D. Blackwell Science. Oxford 1999.

QUESTION   18

A. TRUE   B. TRUE   C. FALSE   D. FALSE   E. TRUE

With any tube inserted into the oesophagus and stomach, only the gastric balloon should be inflated as the flow is from the gastric fundus up the oesophagus. Oesophageal pressure necrosis may otherwise result, and bleeding from fundal varices will be made worse. A Linton tube may be used which only has a gastric balloon. Whereas lactulose may still play a part in removal of blood from the GI tract, there is not considered any place for the use of gut sterilisation now to prevent or diminish hepatic encephalopathy. The synthetic analogue of vasopressin, octreotide is useful in selectively decreasing splanchnic blood flow and portal pressure, at a dose of 3-5 μg/kg/hour. Its use has also been described in other GI bleeding conditions as a temporising measure.

Ref: Shepherd R. Chapter 11. In: *Diseases of the liver and biliary system in childhood*. Ed Kelly D. Blackwell Science. Oxford 1999.

QUESTION 19

A. TRUE   B. FALSE   C. TRUE   D. TRUE   E. FALSE

Even if small amounts of urobilinogen are seen in the urine (usually with unconjugated hyperbilirubinaemia), in biliary atresia this is not usually manifest until after the first day of life. The Kasai procedure is effective whether the biliary atresia is intra or extra-hepatic.

Ref: Roberts E. Chapter 2. In: *Diseases of the liver and biliary system in childhood*. Ed Kelly D. Blackwell Science. Oxford 1999.

QUESTION 20

A. FALSE   B. FALSE   C. FALSE   D. FALSE   E. TRUE

Haemorrhagic disease of the newborn is seen in infants usually during the first week of life, however a late presenting form exists, occurring at around 4-6 weeks. The disease occurs due to a deficiency of Vitamin K-dependent clotting factors, which are a result of an immature gut and low gut bacteria levels. Breast fed babies are at increased risk, as this is a poor source of Vitamin K compared to bottle fed babies. Prophylactic Vitamin K is recommended to be given to all newborn babies to prevent this disease, which is unpredictable. Vitamin K is recommended as an intramuscular dose, though it can be given orally. Bleeding is usually mild but may be catastrophic and fatal. Management is with intravenous vitamin K, FFP, blood and plasma as needed. All liver enzyme inducers taken by the mother will increase the risk of haemorrhagic disease of the newborn.

QUESTION 21

A. TRUE   B. TRUE   C. FALSE   D. FALSE   E. TRUE

Glucose-6-phosphate dehydrogenase (G6PD) deficiency is an X-linked disease, however females may be mildly clinically affected. G6PD is an enzyme involved in the Hexose-Monophosphate shunt (Emden-Meyerhof pathway is affected in pyruvate kinase deficiency). This enzyme deficiency results in the RBC being susceptible to acute haemolysis with oxidant stress. Oxidant stresses include sepsis, drugs (e.g. antimalarials, aspirin, sulphonamides), fava beans (in type B only). Haemolytic crises involve a rapidly developing intravascular haemolysis. Type A (African) is milder as the younger RBCs have normal enzyme activity. Type B (Mediterranean) is more severe as all RBCs are affected.

During a crisis bite cells, blister cells, Heinz bodies, reticulocytes and features of intravascular haemolysis are present.

QUESTION 22

A. FALSE   B. TRUE   C. FALSE   D. TRUE   E. TRUE

In β-thalassaemia major there are reduced or small amounts of beta chains. There are massively increased amounts of foetal haemoglobin (0-70%). A severe anaemia develops from 3-6 months of age when the switch normally occurs from α-chain to β-chain synthesis. Golf-ball cells are due to aggreagates of β-globin chains and are seen in HbH disease. The skull X-ray is described as a "hair on end" appearance as the skull is thickened due to extramedullary haematopoeisis.

Management is with regular transfusions, folic acid supplements and iron chelation therapy. Splenectomy may be necessary in an older child. Bone marrow transplant is recommended in childhood if there is an unaffected HLA-identical sibling.

QUESTION   23

A. TRUE   B. FALSE   C. FALSE   D. TRUE   E. FALSE

In haemophilia A (Classical haemophilia) factor VIII levels are low or absent.

Blood coagulation investigations show a prolonged APTT but normal prothrombin time. Factor VIII activity is reduced.

Management is with prophylactic recombinant factor VIII therapy, and infusions of factor VIII after injury. DDAVP may be used in mild disease to cause a rise in the patient's own factor VIII levels. Antibodies to factor VIII do develop in around 10% of patients.

Methods of carrier detection among females include measuring factor VIII activity which is usually below half of normal. DNA probes provide a more accurate method of diagnosis.

QUESTION   24

A. FALSE   B. TRUE   C. FALSE   D. FALSE   E. TRUE

Vincristine is one of the vinca alkaloids and acts by inhibiting microtubule formation. (Methotrexate is a folic acid antagonist, and the effects can be reversed with folinic acid, not vitamin B6.) Side effects include peripheral neuropathy and SIADH. Other side effects are constipation, jaw pain and seizures. Severe extravasation injuries can occur as it is extremely toxic to tissues. Lung fibrosis may be caused by bleomycin and cyclophosphamide.

QUESTION   25

A. FALSE   B. FALSE   C. FALSE   D. TRUE   E. FALSE

Retinoblastoma may be sporadic or hereditary. The hereditary form is associated with deletions of the long arm (not the short arm) of chromosome 13. Most hereditary tumours are bilateral, but around a fifth are unilateral. The bilateral tumours are diagnosed, on average, earlier than the unilateral tumours. Management may be with radiotherapy to save the eye. Enucleation is only performed when it is unavoidable. These hereditary tumours are associated particularly with secondary osteosarcomas.

QUESTION   26

A. FALSE   B. TRUE   C. FALSE   D. FALSE   E. FALSE

IgE is present in the serum as a monomer and is not divided into subclasses. It interacts with mast cells and basophils via the FcεR1 receptor, resulting in the release of histamine and other mediators, as part of the type 1 hypersensitivity reaction. Levels of IgE are very high in the hyper IgE syndrome, but high levels are not diagnostic of this condition, as they may be found in atopic disease.

Ref. Roitt, Brostoff, Male, Ch 6 In: *Immunology, Fifth Edition*, Mosby, London, 1998. p.73–79

QUESTION 27

A. TRUE   B. FALSE   C. TRUE   D. FALSE   E. FALSE

The DiGeorge anomaly is caused by a microdeletion of chromosome 22q11. It is an autosomal dominant condition. The abnormality causes a failure of development of the 4th branchial arch and this results in the clinical features.

The clinical features are thymus aplasia or hypoplasia which causes the immune defects, hypoparathyroidism, right-sided cardiac defects, oesophageal atresia and facial dysmorphism.

The immune defects are predominantly T cell, with decreased numbers and function of T cells. There may also be specific antibody deficiency and reduced PHA. The immunodeficiency results in recurrent infections with bacteria, fungi and viruses. The severity of these infections is variable and they are not usually the presenting feature.

QUESTION 28

A. FALSE   B. TRUE   C. TRUE   D. TRUE   E. FALSE

Chronic granulomatous disease may be autosomal recessive (33%), or X-linked recessive (66%). The defect is of neutrophil chemotaxis, due to a failure in superoxide production.

Clinical features include granulomas in the gut, liver, spleen, lungs and bone. There are recurrent abscesses in the bones, lungs, liver, gut and lymph nodes. There may also be gingival hyperplasia.

QUESTION 29

A. TRUE   B. FALSE   C. TRUE   D. TRUE   E. FALSE

Measles, BCG and yellow fever vaccines are live-attenuated.

Pertussis contains killed organisms. Influenza contains immunising components of the organisms.

QUESTION 30

A. TRUE   B. FALSE   C. TRUE   D. FALSE   E. TRUE

Toxic shock syndrome is due to *Staphylococcus aureus* phage group I and the clinical features are due to the toxic shock syndrome toxin-1 (TSST-1). A similar clinical syndrome is caused by Group A streptococcus. There is a high fever, hypotension and a rash, and multisystem involvement (with signs of involvement in 3 or more systems being part of the CDC diagnostic criteria). There is almost always diarrhoea and myalgia, the latter resulting in a raised creatinine kinase. Treatment is supportive and with antibiotic therapy.

QUESTION 31

A. FALSE   B. FALSE   C. TRUE   D. TRUE   E. TRUE

Enterobius vermiculata is a threadworm and is a common infection in children. It may be asymptomatic or cause pruritis ani. It may be diagnosed using the Sellotape test. It is treated with piperazine.

QUESTION 32

A. TRUE   B. TRUE   C. TRUE   D. TRUE   E. TRUE

Varicella is highly infectious by personal contact and droplet spread, and the incidence is seasonal. The infectious period (from 2 days before the rash until all the vesicles are dry) may be extended in the immunocompromised patient. Children may develop zoster infection (shingles), though it is more common in the elderly. Immunocompromised children are at more risk of shingles. Zoster in an exposed site (e.g. ophthalmic area) is almost as infectious as chicken pox. Cases of neonatal chicken pox, some of which may be fatal, have been reported despite VZIG prophylaxis.

QUESTION 33

A. FALSE   B. FALSE   C. FALSE   D. FALSE   E. FALSE

Phenylketonuria has an incidence of approximately 1 in 10 000-20 000. It results from a deficiency or absence of the enzyme phenylalanine hydroxylase. This results in an accumulation of phenylalanine and its metabolites, as it is unable to be converted to tyrosine. Converting tyrosine to dopamine is the next step in the pathway. Blood phenylalanine levels are only raised after protein feeds begin. This is the reason that the Guthrie test must be done at least 24-48 hours after birth, to avoid false negatives (the Guthrie test detects blood phenylalanine levels). The classical features of fair hair and skin and blue eyes are only seen when the condition is not treated, and thus they should rarely be seen in the UK now. Management is a diet low in phenylalanine which is now recommended for life. A small amount of phenylalanine needs to be given as it cannot be synthesised by the body. The diet is particularly important during pregnancy, as high phenylalanine levels are toxic to the foetus and result in abnormalities.

QUESTION 34

A. TRUE   B. FALSE   C. TRUE   D. FALSE   E. TRUE

Pompe disease is one of the glycogen storage diseases (GSD 2). It classically involves a cardiomyopathy, skeletal muscle myopathy, macroglossia and early death. A late form does exist which presents as a myopathy. The enzyme deficiency is acid maltase.

There are 9 different glycogen storage diseases, and Pompe disease is one of the commonest. Both GSD 1 and GSD 3 include hepatomegaly and hypoglycaemia and continuous overnight feeds are necessary to avoid complications.

Diagnosis is by enzyme analysis in blood, liver or muscle biopsy.

QUESTION 35

A. TRUE   B. FALSE   C. TRUE   D. TRUE   E. TRUE

Hepatorenal tyrosinaemia is a result of the enzyme deficiency of fumarylacetoacetase. There is resulting tyrosinaemia and succinylacetonuria. It is associated with French-Canadians (Quebecois). The main features are of renal Fanconi syndrome and hepatocellular degeneration.

Diagnosis is by enzyme analysis in cultured fibroblasts, plasma amino acid profile (tyrosine elevated) and urine organic acid profile (succinylacetone elevated). Serum α-FP is raised and liver biopsy shows features of cirrhosis.

Management is with a low tyrosine and phenylalanine diet. NTBC therapy, which acts essentially by turning tyrosinaemia type 1 into the more benign tyrosinaemia type 2 is also used. Liver transplant early in the disease is the definitive therapy.

QUESTION 36

A. FALSE   B. FALSE   C. FALSE   D. FALSE   E. TRUE

In normal puberty in boys, the first sign is testicular enlargement, with a testicular volume of 4 ml indicating the onset of puberty. Onset of puberty in boys ranges from 9-14 years, with an average age of 11.8 years. The pubertal growth spurt occurs later at around 13.9 years. Early (precocious) puberty is most often pathological in boys.

QUESTION 37

A. FALSE   B. FALSE   C. TRUE   D. TRUE   E. FALSE

The classical features of neonatal hyperthyroidism include:

- Prematurity and IUGR
- Neonatal jaundice, microcephaly, exophthalmos and goitre
- Tachycardia, tachpnoea, hyperthermia and hypertension

QUESTION 38

A. TRUE   B. FALSE   C. TRUE   D. TRUE   E. TRUE

Hyponatraemia as a part of SIADH (syndrome of inappropriate ADH secretion) may result from many causes. These include the drugs carbamazepine and cyclophosphamide. Glibenclamide can cause diabetes insipidus. Both cystic fibrosis and Ewing's sarcoma can cause SIADH. The causes of SIADH can be divided for simplicity into cranial (e.g. brain abscess, meningitis), tumours, lungs (e.g. pneumonia), metabolic (e.g. acute interittent porphyria) and drugs.

QUESTION 39

A. FALSE   B. FALSE   C. FALSE   D. TRUE   E. TRUE

In congenital adrenal hyperplasia of the most common type (due to 21-hydroxylase deficiency), there are elevated plasma levels of potassium, ACTH, testosterone, androstenedione and 17-hydroxyprogesterone.

There are decreased levels of plasma sodium, glucose, cortisol and aldosterone.

QUESTION 40

A. TRUE   B. TRUE   C. FALSE   D. FALSE   E. FALSE

The facial nerve has both motor and sensory components. It supplies the muscles of facial expression and has secretomotor fibres to the lachrymal gland and to the submandibular and sublingual salivary glands. It also transmits taste fibres from the anterior two thirds of the tongue. There are separate pontine nuclei for each of these three functions. The motor nucleus is in the reticular formation of the lower pons.

The course of the facial nerve runs from the lower border of the pons into the internal auditory meatus with the auditory nerve, and then into the facial canal. The facial nerve then passes through the stylomastoid foramen. All the sensory components have left by the time the nerve emerges through the stylomastoid foramen.

A unilateral lesion of the motor nucleus will affect the lower part of the contralateral face only. This is because the upper part of the nucleus which controls the lower facial muscles receives only contralateral fibres, whereas the lower part of the nucleus (which controls the upper facial muscles) receives both crossed and uncrossed fibres.

QUESTION   41

A. TRUE   B. FALSE   C. TRUE   D. TRUE   E. FALSE

At 18 months, children should have around 6 words. Echolalia is a normal language deviation in children under 2.5 years. Hand dominance under 1 year may be a sign of brain damage. Pincer grasp should develop from 9 months. Bottom shuffling is a normal variant, and these children usually walk late, on average at around 22 months.

QUESTION   42

A. FALSE   B. FALSE   C. TRUE   D. TRUE   E. FALSE

Lennox-Gastaut syndrome has an onset between 3-10 years, mostly occurring at 4-5 years. It is a clinico-electric syndrome of several types of seizures and an EEG pattern of slow spike and wave forms. Loss of language skills and seizures is seen in the Landau-Kleffner syndrome. Approximately 50% of children with intractable epilepsy have Lennox-Gastuat syndrome. There is mental handicap in most children prior to onset of the seizures, and there is then further deterioration.

QUESTION   43

A. FALSE   B. FALSE   C. TRUE   D. TRUE   E. FALSE

Myotonic dystrophy is a disease of progressive proximal muscle weakness with failure of muscle relaxation. The heart may be affected with conduction defects and cardiomyopathy. There are learning difficulties in around 50% of affected individuals. There is frontal baldness in males, and cataracts are commonly seen. Muscle biopsy is used in diagnosis. Children born to carrier mothers are more severely affected.

QUESTION   44

A. TRUE   B. TRUE   C. TRUE   D. TRUE   E. TRUE

They may all present as an acute abdomen. There are many non-surgical causes of acute abdomen, including:

Urinary tract infection, pneumonia, diabetic ketoacidosis, Henoch-Schönlein purpura, acute viral hepatits, a sickle cell disease crisis and a haemolytic episode in congenital spherocytosis.

QUESTION   45

A. TRUE   B. FALSE   C. TRUE   D. FALSE   E. FALSE

Vigabatrin may cause a dose-related depression or psychosis. Vigabatrin has been used as first line treatment in infantile spasms. It is contraindicated in generalised tonic clonic seizures as it may make these worse. Visual field defects are seen in up to 40% of adults with long term use, most cases being asymptomatic.

QUESTION   46

A. FALSE   B. TRUE   C. FALSE   D. FALSE   E. TRUE

Frusemide is both rapid in onset and short-acting. It results in hypokalaemia as a result of the Na^+-K^+ pump activation in the distal renal tubule. Nephrocalcinosis can occur in neonates as calcium is excreted from the tubules.

QUESTION 47

A. TRUE   B. TRUE   C. FALSE   D. TRUE   E. FALSE

Erythromycin is bacteriostatic, but the newer macrolides can be bacteriocidal in high concentration. Erythromycin increases interdigestive (but not post-prandial) gastric and duodenal motility. Cholestatic hepatitis may occur and is more likely with erythromycin than the newer macrolide antibiotics (e.g. azithromycin or clarithromycin). Both terfinadine and astemizole should be avoided with macrolide antibiotics due to the risk of serious cardiac arrhythmia.

QUESTION 48

A. TRUE   B. TRUE   C. FALSE   D. FALSE   E. FALSE

Allopurinol inhibits azathioprine metabolism, and thus the risk of bone marrow suppression is increased.

Sodium valproate is a liver enzyme inhibitor, unlike other anticonvulsants which are liver enzyme inducers.

Griseofulvin is a liver enzyme inducer.

In slow acetylators the standard dose of isoniazid interferes with pyridoxine metabolism, increasing the risk of neuropathy.

A reduction in bacterial vitamin K synthesis in the large bowel may potentiate the effects of warfarin.

QUESTION 49

A. TRUE   B. TRUE   C. TRUE   D. TRUE   E. TRUE

Erythema multiforme is a skin reaction which may be induced by infections, drugs and other causes (see below). It appears as symmetrical erythematous lesions, occurring in crops. The rash may become bullous. Target lesions are seen (red border, dusky centre, with pale ring in between).

Causes include infections such as HSV (commonly) and *Mycoplasma pneumoniae* and drugs such as sulphonamides. Other causes include leukaemia and lymphoma.

Stevens-Johnson syndrome is thought to represent a severe form of the disease with mucous membrane involvement (oral and genital ulcers) and constitutional disturbance.

QUESTION 50

A. FALSE   B. TRUE   C. TRUE   D. FALSE   E. TRUE

Rheumatoid factor is an antibody to the Fc portion of IgG. It may be positive in JCA, rheumatoid arthritis, SLE, Sjögren's syndrome, chronic infections (e.g. HIV, TB, endocarditis, hepatitis), lymphoid malignancies, leukaemia and pulmonary fibrosis.

Anti-centromere antibody is one of the antinuclear antibodies (ANA) and is seen in CREST syndrome. Other ANA antibodies are anti-ds DNA (SLE, 80%, specific), anti-ss DNA (SLE, 90%, non-specific, other connective tissue diseases) and anti-histone (SLE, particularly drug-induced lupus).

Anti-neutrophil cytoplasmic antibodies (ANCA) are: c-ANCA (cytoplasmic) which is specific to Wegener's granulomatosis, and p-ANCA (perinuclear) which is seen in vasculitis and connective tissue diseases.

QUESTION 51

A. TRUE   B. FALSE   C. TRUE   D. TRUE   E. FALSE

Subcutaneous nodules are found in a number of diseases including:

- Churg–Strauss syndrome
- RhF positive polyarticular JCA
- Rheumatic fever
- Scleroderma (tendon nodules)

QUESTION 52

A. TRUE   B. FALSE   C. FALSE   D. TRUE   E. TRUE

Amyloidosis is a disease involving deposition of amyloid in the extracellular matrix. It may be primary or secondary.

Primary amyloidosis is associated with myeloma and macroglobulinaemia.

Secondary amyloidosis is associated with systemic JCA, Familial Mediterranean fever and inflammatory bowel disease.

Nephrotic syndrome is a feature of secondary amyloidosis.

Biopsy of affected tissue is stained with Congo red, but is green under polarising light. The amyloid in secondary amyloidosis is a unique protein (AA), but in primary disease it is homologous with immunoglobulin κ or λ light chains (AL).

Treatment is that of the underlying disease. Alkylating agents may be used in secondary amyloid.

QUESTION 53

A. FALSE   B. FALSE   C. FALSE   D. FALSE   E. TRUE

As a general rule, autosomal recessive conditions are frequently metabolic disorders, and autosomal dominant disorders are often structural defects.

Klinefelter syndrome (47, XXY) is a chromosomal abnormality affecting approximately 1 in 500 males.

Duchenne muscular dystrophy is an X-linked recessive condition, with mutations in the DMD gene encoding for the protein dystrophin.

Familial hypophosphataemic rickets is an X-linked dominant condition.

Marfan's syndrome is an autosomal dominant condition resulting from mutations in the fibrillin gene (FBN1) on chromosome 15q21.1.

Homocystinuria is an autosomal recessively inherited condition caused by an enzyme deficiency of cystathione synthase resulting in homocystine and methionine accumulation.

QUESTION 54

A. FALSE   B. FALSE   C. FALSE   D. TRUE   E. FALSE

CHARGE association stands for Coloboma, Heart disease, Atresia choanae, Retarded growth and development, Genital anomalies and Ear anomalies. Cardiac defects associated are tetralogy of Fallot, patent ductus arteriosus, VSD, ASD, right sided aortic arch and double outlet right ventricle with an atrioventricular canal defect.

Neurofibromatosis is associated with pulmonary stenosis and coarctation of the aorta.

Holt-Oram syndrome includes a secundum ASD or VSD associated with radial aplasia.

Chromosome 22 microdeletion is associated with aortic arch anomalies (e.g. right sided aortic arch, interrupted aorta), truncus arteriosus, VSD, PDA and Tetralogy of Fallot.

Hunter syndrome is associated with aortic regurgitation and mitral regurgitation.

QUESTION 55

A. FALSE   B. TRUE   C. FALSE   D. FALSE   E. TRUE

The heart is formed from mesoderm tissue, and develops as a primitive heart tube. This tube is forced to bend as it develops. The descending limb of the loop becomes the left ventricle, and the ascending limb (the bulbus cordis) forms part of the right ventricle. The cardiac chambers are formed by the end of the 4th week, and the heart begins to beat at around 23 days.

The first, second and fifth aortic arches disappear. The third arch gives rise to the bifurcation of the internal and external carotids. The left fourth arch gives rise to the arch of the aorta. The right fourth arch develops into the right subclavian artery. The sixth aortic arch develops into the pulmonary arteries, with the ductus arteriosus forming from the remnant of the sixth right aortic arch.

QUESTION 56

A. TRUE   B. FALSE   C. FALSE   D. TRUE   E. FALSE

In a Normal distribution the mode, median and mean are equal.

The standard deviation is a measure of how the values are scattered on either side of the mean. 68% of the values will lie within +/- one standard deviation of the mean. The standard error of the mean is calculated by dividing the standard deviation of the sample by the square root of the sample size.

QUESTION 57

A. FALSE   B. FALSE   C. TRUE   D. TRUE   E. FALSE

Neonatal mortality rate is the number of deaths of liveborn infants within 28 days of birth per 1000 live births.

Infant mortality rate is the number of deaths between birth and 1 year per 1000 live births.

Perinatal mortality rate is the number of stillbirths plus deaths within the first 6 days per 1000 births (live and still).

This stillbirth rate is the number of stillbirths per 1000 of all births (live and still).

A neonate is an infant below 28 days old.

QUESTION 58

A. TRUE   B. FALSE   C. TRUE   D. FALSE   E. TRUE

Umbilical hernia in infancy is more common in African infants. It is also seen in Beckwith-Weidemann syndrome, hypothyroidism and is more common in premature infants.

QUESTION 59

A. FALSE   B. FALSE   C. TRUE   D. TRUE   E. TRUE

Maternal α-fetoprotein levels are decreased in Trisomy 18, Trisomy 21 and intrauterine growth retardation. Levels of α-fetoprotein are increased in epidermolysis bullosa, multiple pregnancy and cystic hygroma. Other causes of increased levels are foeto-maternal haemorrhage, anencephaly, open spina bifida, anterior abdominal wall defects and polycystic kidney disease.

QUESTION 60

A. TRUE   B. FALSE   C. TRUE   D. TRUE   E. FALSE

The mean airway pressure is the average pressure to which the lungs are expanded during the respiratory cycle. An increase in the gas flow rate does not affect the pCO_2, though it can increase the pO_2.

A high PEEP can impede CO_2 elimination because it decreases the tidal volume.

An increase in PIP will cause a fall in the pCO_2 and a rise in the pO_2.

The pO_2 is the partial pressure of oxygen in equilibrium with blood. The percentage haemoglobin bound with oxygen at a given pO_2 is the oxygen saturation.

Exam 2: Questions

QUESTION 1

Physiological (innocent) murmurs

A. Are heard in a small minority of children
B. May have a diastolic component
C. Characteristically change in intensity with the position of the patient
D. Are more common in infants who are small for their gestational age
E. May be associated with a thrill

QUESTION 2

Regarding coarctation of the aorta

A. It may present with circulatory collapse in neonates
B. The post-operative re-coarctation rate is approximately 20%
C. It usually occurs just proximally to the origin of the left subclavian artery
D. Rib notching is usually present by 4 years af age
E. It is associated with Berry aneurysm

QUESTION 3

The following are major Duckett-Jones criteria for the diagnosis of rheumatic fever

A. Arthralgia
B. Pericarditis
C. Subcutaneous nodules
D. Huntington's chorea
E. Erythema nodosum

QUESTION 4

Ebstein's anomaly

A. Gives rise to a soft systolic murmer
B. May be asymptomatic
C. Is associated with Wolff-Parkinson-White syndrome type A
D. Involves a distal displacement of the mitral valve
E. Results in massive cardiomegaly on the chest X-ray

QUESTION   5

The following are correct

A. The total lung capacity is increased in asthma
B. There is a low FEV1:FVC ratio in restrictive lung disease
C. Sarcoidosis is a restrictive airway disease
D. Surfactant causes a fall in lung compliance
E. Hyperkinetic states can cause a high transfer factor for carbon monoxide

QUESTION   6

The following are true of chemotherapy for tuberculosis

A. Visual acuity assessment is necessary prior to commencing pyrazinamide
B. Ethambutol should be avoided in young children
C. Psychosis may occur with isoniazid therapy secondary to nicotinamide deficiency
D. Rifampicin has increased side-effects in slow acetylators
E. Chemoprophylaxis should be given to infants with a positive Mantoux test

QUESTION   7

Regarding lung function tests in pre-school children

A. Tidal flow-volume loop technique uses a ratio of time needed to reach maximum flow versus total expiratory time as an index of total resistance of the airways
B. The forced oscillation technique is non-invasive but requires acceptance of a closely fitting mask and only tidal breathing
C. Whole body plethysmography is regarded as the 'gold standard' for lung function measurements in young children
D. The interrupter technique is generally non-variable and easily reproducible
E. Transcutaneous oxygen measurement in asthma reflects relatively accurately the clinical state of the patient

QUESTION   8

In an infant with gastro-oesophageal reflux

A. A reflux index (time below pH 4) of 8% is considered to lie within the normal range
B. Sudden infant death syndrome is a recognised sequela
C. Due to cow's milk sensitivity, the milk of choice is soya-based
D. An examination of a bag urine or MSU is not necessary
E. There is a 90-95% chance of complete resolution by 2 years of age

QUESTION 9

Schwachman-Diamond syndrome

A. Can involve red cell aplasia
B. Can reveal a high HbF on electropheresis
C. Can involve epiphyseal dysostosis
D. Progression to myeloid arrest can occur
E. Average survival is approximately 15 years

QUESTION 10

If a polyp or polyps are present in the colon of a 12 year old boy

A. Painful bright red bleeding with autolysis is the most common presentation
B. Retinal pigmentation is an early clinical marker for familial adenomatous polyposis coli
C. Mucosal pigmentation around the mouth indicates that there is a 50% chance of him developing malignant tumours outside the GI tract
D. And are seen by barium follow through, then ulcerative colitis is a possible diagnosis
E. Recurrent volvulus is likely after 1 year if removal is not undertaken

QUESTION 11

In children with diseases affecting the oral cavity

A. Swelling of the lips may be the sole manifestation of Crohn's disease
B. Oral ulceration can be demonstrated in 60% of those with Behçet's disease
C. Recurrent aphthous ulceration is usually due to cyclical neutropaenia
D. Ulcers due to tuberculosis are in most cases secondary to pulmonary disease
E. Gum hypertrophy may be a manifestation of acrodermatitis enteropathica

QUESTION 12

The following are true of renal function in neonates

A. Polycythaemia may cause renal vein thrombosis
B. Renal blood flow is high and resistance low at birth
C. Renal tubular function may be poor in the first week
D. Glomerular filtration rate attains adult levels by approximately 4 months of age
E. Irreversible renal damage may have occurred by the time of birth in males with posterior urethral valve obstruction

QUESTION   13

Renal calculi

A. Secondary to ileostomies, will consist primarily of calcium phosphate

B. Which are termed 'staghorn' are secondary to urease-splitting organisms

C. May result from cytinosis

D. May result from xanthinuria

E. Occur in proximal renal tubular acidosis, whereas nephrocalcinosis occurs with distal renal tubular acidosis

QUESTION   14

Typically haemolytic uraemic syndrome

A. Is associated with *Shigella*

B. Is familial

C. Causes death mainly by hypokalaemia

D. Presenting with a high white cell count is associated with a worse prognosis

E. Features an abnormal coagulation screen

QUESTION   15

Features which distinguish renal from pre-renal failure include

A. Urine:plasma osmolality ratio < 1.2

B. Mean arterial blood pressure > 95

C. Urine specific gravity > 1020

D. Urinary sodium > 15 mmol/l

E. Hyperkalaemia

QUESTION   16

The following are recognised causes of cirrhosis in childhood

A. Post-bone marrow transplant veno-occlusive disease

B. Alpha-1 anti-trypsin genotype PiMS

C. Acute viral hepatitis

D. Autoimmune hepatitis with liver-kidney-microsomal antibody positivity

E. Extra-hepatic biliary atresia with Kasai performed at 80 days of age

QUESTION   17

Hepatitis A

A. Is infective until just after jaundice appears

B. Can be associated with a Coomb's positive haemolytic anaemia

C. Can be diagnosed by the finding on electron microscopy of viral particles in the faeces

D. Has a 10% chance of subsequent hepatocellular carcinoma in the 30 years following infection

E. Is caused by a DNA hepadna virus

QUESTION   18

In paediatric orthotopic liver transplant

- **A.** Generalised mitochondrial cytopathy is a recognised indication
- **B.** The major indication in Alagille's syndrome is deteriorating liver synthetic function
- **C.** The host liver is left in situ
- **D.** CMV status of host and recipient is unimportant
- **E.** 5 year survival rate for an elective transplant is 80–90%

QUESTION   19

When liver pathology is responsible for an acutely ill baby

- **A.** Intraocular 'oildrop' cataracts point towards galactosaemia as the diagnosis
- **B.** Blood and urine should always be taken and stored at -70 °C if hypoglycaemia is present
- **C.** Hyperlactataemia excludes mitochondrial cytopathies
- **D.** Bile-stained vomiting points towards biliary atresia
- **E.** Intragastric infusion of ursodeoxycholic acid is important in the initial management

QUESTION   20

The following result in a shift of the oxy-haemoglobin dissociation curve to the right

- **A.** Acute alkalosis
- **B.** Fever
- **C.** A fall in 2,3 DPG
- **D.** Methaemoglobin
- **E.** Fetal haemoglobin

QUESTION   21

Pyruvate kinase deficiency

- **A.** Is X-linked and females may be mildly affected
- **B.** Is more common than G6PD deficiency
- **C.** Prickle cells are seen in the blood film
- **D.** Splenectomy may result in massive reticulocytosis
- **E.** The symptoms of anaemia are milder than expected for the haemoglobin level

QUESTION   22

In hereditary spherocytosis

- **A.** Anaemia is always present
- **B.** The disease is due to a defect in ankyrin
- **C.** Aplastic crises may occur with parvovirus infection
- **D.** Neonatal jaundice may be severe enough to cause kernicterus
- **E.** Inheritance is autosomal recessive

QUESTION   23

Regarding von Willebrand disease

A. The disease is more severe in males
B. von Willebrand factor promotes platelet adhesion
C. The disease shows variable expression
D. The bleeding time is usually normal
E. Platelets are large

QUESTION   24

Regarding acute graft-versus-host disease (GVHD)

A. Donor B lymphocytes mount an immune response to host MHC antigens
B. Cholestatic hepatitis may be a feature
C. Malabsorption may be seen
D. Active malignancy at the time of bone marrow transplantation predisposes to acute GVHD
E. There can be a beneficial effect

QUESTION   25

Regarding brain tumours

A. Posterior fossa tumours are more common than supratentorial tumours in infants under 2 years old
B. Medulloblastoma commonly presents with truncal ataxia
C. Astrocytomas are fast-growing tumours
D. Astrocytomas may be managed solely with resection
E. Brain stem gliomas have a 5 year survival of approximately 60%

QUESTION   26

Selective IgA deficiency

A. May be asymptomatic
B. Has a prevelance in the UK of 1 in 5000
C. Is associated with IgG_1 subclass deficiency
D. Is associated with increased transfusion reactions
E. Is associated with SLE

QUESTION 27

The following are true

A. The Jak 3 mutation is seen in adenosine deaminase deficiency (ADA)
B. Both SCID and HIV infection may present in a similar fashion in an infant
C. The RAG-1 or RAG-2 mutations are seen in purine nucleoside phosphorylase (PNP) deficiency
D. Failure to thrive, diarrhoea and recurrent oral candidiasis in a young infant may be caused by X-linked agammaglobulinaemia
E. Features similar to graft versus host disease may be seen in the neonatal period in an infant with SCID

QUESTION 28

In Chediak–Higashi syndrome

A. Inheritance is X-linked recessive
B. There is abnormal leucocyte adhesion
C. Partial oculocutaneous albinism is a feature
D. Peripheral nerve lesions may be seen
E. EB virus infection can lead to an accelerated phase of disease

QUESTION 29

The following are contraindications to vaccination

A. Previous history of pertussis
B. Family history of adverse reaction following vaccination
C. Over the age recommended in the immunisation schedule
D. Snuffles
E. Cerebral palsy

QUESTION 30

In typhoid fever

A. There is a leucopaenia
B. Rose spots appear on the trunk during the first week of the illness
C. There is a relative bradycardia
D. The second week is the week of complications
E. Blood cultures are 80% positive during the first week

QUESTION   31

Schistisoma haemotobium

A. Is a trematode
B. Commonly causes fibrotic liver disease
C. Is transmitted by tsetse flies
D. Causes Katayama fever
E. Is associated with an increased risk of bladder cancer

QUESTION   32

Parvovirus B19

A. Is the cause of Sixth disease in children
B. Acquired in-utero can result in hydrops foetalis
C. May result in aplastic crises in children with pyruvate kinase deficiency
D. Causes an arthritis most commonly in adults
E. May cause asymptomatic infection

QUESTION   33

Features of homocystinuria include

A. Mental retardation as an uncommon occurrence
B. Upward lens dislocation
C. Arterial and venous thromboembolism
D. Osteoporosis
E. It may be responsive to high dose vitamin B_6 (pyridoxine) therapy

QUESTION   34

Hurler's disease

A. Is a mucopolysaccharidosis
B. Features a clouded cornea
C. Features chondrodysplasia punctata
D. Urine glycosaminoglycans are lowered
E. Is inherited in an X-linked recessive fashion

QUESTION   35

The following disorders are associated with neonatal hypoglycaemia

A. Polycythaemia
B. The organic acidaemias
C. Galactosaemia
D. Glycogen storage disease type 2
E. Down's syndrome

QUESTION 36

During puberty in girls

A. The first sign is the menarche
B. The menarche occurs at an earlier average age in the USA than in the UK
C. The pubertal growth spurt occurs before the menarche
D. The menarche usually occurs at breast stage 2
E. The onset is usually between 7-11 years

QUESTION 37

Hyperthyroidism in children

A. Is usually caused by a solitary adenoma
B. Is more common in males
C. May result in delayed bone age
D. May be associated with HLA B8
E. May be associated with idiopathic thrombocytopaenic purpura

QUESTION 38

The following may help to find the underlying cause of Cushing's syndrome

A. ACTH level
B. Overnight dexamethasone test
C. Adrenal CT scan
D. Urine 24 hour free cortisol
E. High dose dexamethasone test

QUESTION 39

In the syndrome of inappropriate ADH secretion

A. Serum osmolality is high
B. Plasma bicarbonate is high
C. There may be seizures
D. There is peripheral oedema
E. Urine sodium is usually < 20 mmol/day

QUESTION 40

A complete third nerve palsy will result in

A. A partial ptosis
B. Loss of the pupillary light reflex
C. A divergent squint
D. A small irregular pupil
E. Double vision

QUESTION 41

Regarding the primitive reflexes

A. The Moro reflex disappears at 6-8 months
B. The palmar grasp disappears at 9-10 months
C. The stepping reflex may persist in children with cerebral palsy
D. The forward parachute reflex is present from birth
E. The lateral propping reflex develops from around 7 months

QUESTION 42

Infantile spasms

A. Have an onset usually in the neonatal period
B. Usually have no identifiable cause
C. Have an EEG picture of slow spike and wave forms
D. Are always associated with developmental regression
E. May be treated with vigabatrin

QUESTION 43

In Werdnig-Hoffmann disease

A. There is a degeneration of the anterior horn cells
B. The extra-ocular muscles are unaffected
C. The serum creatinine kinase (CK) is elevated
D. Arthrogryphosis may be present
E. There is tongue fasciculation

QUESTION 44

The following are common causes of gastrointestinal bleeding in a neonate

A. Intussuception
B. Henoch-Schönlein purpura
C. Necrotising enterocolitis
D. Polyp
E. Foreign body

QUESTION 45

The following concerning dornase alfa (DNAse) are true

A. It transforms cystic fibrosis sputum from a gel into a flowing liquid in vitro
B. It is ineffective in idiopathic bronchiectasis
C. It is derived from bacterial DNAse
D. It has not been proven to reduce the frequency of respiratory exacerbations in cystic fibrosis
E. It must be given by nebuliser

QUESTION 46

The following concerning analgesia are true

A. Rectal diclofenac improves post-operative pain and reduces opiate requirement
B. Pethidine is recommended for sickle cell crisis pain
C. Morphine is mostly eliminated by the kidneys
D. Fentanyl causes less constipation than morphine
E. Ibuprofen has been shown to have a similar gastric irritant effect to paracetamol

QUESTION 47

The following concerning cephalosporins are true

A. They inhibit bacterial cell wall synthesis
B. Third generation cephalosporins have less activity against gram negative bacteria than the first generation
C. Ceftazidime is less effective against pseudomonas than cefotaxime
D. Patients with penicillin allergy very rarely cross-react with cephalosporins
E. Ceftriaxone has a half-life of less than 2 hours

QUESTION 48

The following are recognised side-effects

A. Hydralazine and drug-induced lupus erythematosis
B. Sodium cromoglycate and diarrhoea
C. Metoclopramide and torticollis
D. Growth hormone and hypothyroidism
E. Ciprofloxacin and arthropathy

QUESTION 49

Regarding the Sturge-Weber syndrome

A. It involves a facial port-wine stain roughly in the distribution of the maxillary and mandibular branches of the trigeminal nerve
B. Glaucoma of the ipsilateral eye is always present
C. MRI brain scan should be performed in the initial investigations
D. It involves a facial capillary haemangioma roughly in the distribution of the ophthalmic and maxillary branches of the trigeminal nerve
E. Surgery may be required to treat resistant seizures

QUESTION 50

Pauciarticular onset juvenile chronic arthritis

A. Includes involvement of 5 or less large joints in the first 6 months of disease
B. Type I is most commonly seen in young females
C. Chronic iridocyclitis occurs in approximately 70% of type I
D. Includes juvenile onset spondyloarthropathy
E. RhF is usually positive

QUESTION 51

Regarding infective arthritis

A. Yersinia infection is more commonly seen in the presence of iron overload
B. It most commonly affects children over 2 years old
C. It may be caused by Guinea worm
D. Joint washout is always necessary in hip disease
E. Pseudoparesis of the affected limb is seen in children

QUESTION 52

Osteogenesis imperfecta

A. Results from a defect in the α-chain of type VII collagen
B. Wormian bones are seen on skull X-ray
C. Type IV disease involves blue sclerae
D. Is always inherited in an autosomal recessive fashion
E. Is associated with a conductive deafness

QUESTION 53

The following are features of Patau syndrome

A. Holoprosencephaly
B. Rocker-bottom feet
C. Scalp defects
D. Patent ductus arteriosus
E. Cryptorchidism

QUESTION 54

The maternal teratogen warfarin is associated with the following congenital defects

A. Neural tube defects
B. Absent thymus
C. Chondrodysplasia punctata
D. Ebstein's anomaly
E. Nasal hypoplasia

QUESTION 55

In the embryological development of the central nervous system

A. The neural plate is derived from endodermal cells
B. The neural tube closes at the end of the fifth week
C. The spinal cord terminates alongside L3 in the newborn
D. The cerebral hemispheres develop from the prosencephalon
E. The pons and cerebellum develop from the diencephalon

QUESTION 56

The following are true

A. In a negatively skewed population, the mean is greater than the mode
B. The null hypothesis assumes there is a significant difference between two populations
C. The variance is the square root of the standard deviation
D. If an assay is 100% specific, there may be false positives
E. The t-test may be used on non-parametric data

QUESTION 57

Regarding antenatal diagnosis

A. The triple test for Down's syndrome includes serum αFP, serum HCG and serum uE3
B. Nuchal fold thickness is measured to screen for Down's syndrome at 8-12 weeks
C. Amniocentesis carries a 1:1000 risk of miscarriage
D. Chorionic villous sampling may be done at around 12 weeks
E. Gestational age estimate by ultrasound is reliable if done prior to 28 weeks

QUESTION 58

Respiratory distress syndrome

A. May be prevented by antenatal steroids
B. Is more common in infants of diabetic mothers
C. Is more common in the second of twins
D. Is more likely if there is a high lecithin:sphingomyelin ratio
E. Is more common in infants with intrauterine growth retardation (IUGR)

QUESTION 59

Regarding gastroschisis and omphalocoele

A. Gastroschisis is more common then omphalocoele
B. Herniation of the liver is common in omphalocoele
C. Extraintestinal abnormalities are commonly associated with gastroschisis
D. Chromosomal anomalies are seen commonly with omphalocoele
E. The defect in gastroschisis occurs at the left paraumbilial area

QUESTION 60

Polyhydramnios is associated with the following

A. VACTERL association
B. Maternal diabetes
C. Infantile polycystic kidney disease
D. Potter syndrome
E. Congenital myotonic dystrophy

Exam 2: Answers

QUESTION 1

A. FALSE B. TRUE C. TRUE D. FALSE E. FALSE

Physiological murmurs are common, being heard in approximately 30% of children. They are of two types:

1. Ejection murmurs due to turbulent flow in the outflow tracts from the heart.
2. Venous hum due to turbulent flow in the head and neck veins.

They have certain characteristics that help identify them as innocent murmurs. These include:-

Usually soft (grade 2 or below), usually systolic (though venous hum is a continuous low pitched rumble). The heart sounds are normal and there is no radiation of the murmur or associated thrill. They do change with altered position, and also with exercise. The patient is asymptomatic with normal pulses, and the ECG and CXR are normal.

QUESTION 2

A. TRUE B. FALSE C. FALSE D. FALSE E. TRUE

Coarctation of the aorta is a constriction of the aorta, usually occurring just distal to the origin of the left subclavian artery. It may present in the neonatal period as collapse in the first week. Late presentation may be with discovery of a murmur or absent femoral pulses, as hypertension or as heart failure.

Rib-notching is not usually present until over the age of 8 years, and occurs due to the development of collaterals beneath the ribs. Berry aneurysms are associated. Other associations are Turner's syndrome, a VSD and mitral valve anomalies. A biscuspid aortic valve is present in about 40% of cases.

Surgical repair is necessary, and the recoarctation rate is around 5%.

QUESTION 3

A. FALSE B. TRUE C. TRUE D. FALSE E. FALSE

The Duckett-Jones criteria for diagnosing rheumatic fever include major and minor criteria.

Two major and two minor criteria are needed to make the diagnosis.

The major criteria are:

- Carditis (endocarditis, myocarditis and/or pericarditis)
- Polyarthritis
- Sydenham's chorea
- Erythema marginatum
- Subcutaneous nodules

Minor criteria are fever, arthralgia, leucocytosis, a raised ESR or CRP, a long P-R interval and previous rheumatic fever.

Huntington's chorea is an inherited condition with premature onset of dementia and death.

QUESTION 4

A. TRUE   B. TRUE   C. FALSE   D. FALSE   E. TRUE

Ebstein's anomaly involves an abnormal tricuspid valve with distal displacement of the tricuspid valve and atrialization of the right ventricle. There is an ASD and functional pulmonary atresia. Wolf-Parkinson White syndrome type B is associated.

Clinical features are cyanosis and failure to thrive. Arrhthymias occur with extrasystoles and SVTs. It may be asymptomatic as the anatomical abnormalities are of varying severity.

There is a soft, long systolic murmur due to tricuspid regurgitation. There are also diastolic murmurs and extra heart sounds.

The CXR shows a massive cardiomegaly and pulmonary oligaemia, though it may be normal.

QUESTION 5

A. TRUE   B. FALSE   C. TRUE   D. FALSE   E. TRUE

The total lung capacity is increased in asthma, but the FVC is decreased due to air trapping (and the residual volume is therefore increased).

Restrictive lung disease causes a fall in both the FVC and the FEV1, and so the ratio is normal or even slightly increased.

Sarcoidosis produces a restrictive airway disease.

Surfactant increases lung compliance.

The transfer factor for carbon monoxide is increased in hyperkinetic states as there is increased pulmonary blood flow.

QUESTION 6

A. FALSE   B. TRUE   C. FALSE   D. FALSE   E. TRUE

Visual acuity assessment should be done prior to commencing ethambutol as it can cause blurred vision, scotoma and colour blindness. For this reason, ethambutol should be avoided in young children as they cannot report visual disturbance.

Isoniazid therapy can cause a psychosis, but it is secondary to pyridoxine deficiency.

Isoniazid produces increased effects in slow acetylators. Infants with a positive Mantoux test should be given 6-9 months of chemoprophylaxis with isoniazid.

QUESTION 7

A. TRUE   B. TRUE   C. TRUE   D. FALSE   E. TRUE

In airway obstruction, the total time for expiration increases while the time to reach maximal flow decreases, thus decreasing the ratio. It requires validation in younger children.

In the forced oscillation technique, a sound source generates a pressure pulse every 3 seconds which passes via the tubing and mask into the airways. These are reflected back as resonance, consisting of flow, which is measured by flow detectors and related to pressure changes measured by pressure transducers, thus estimating impedance.

There are many variables in the interrupter technique that can be altered, making it an inconsistent method for measuring resistance.

Transcutaneous oxygen measurement reflects V:Q mismatch rather than lung function, though it does reflect the clinical state of the patient.

QUESTION 8

A. TRUE   B. TRUE   C. FALSE   D. FALSE   E. TRUE

A reflux index less than 10% in infancy and less than 6% thereafter is still considered 'normal', although it must be stressed that the trace and event markers must be looked at and correlated. Substitution with a cow's milk hydrolysate milk is the milk of choice (e.g. Pregestimil, Nutramigen, Peptijunior, or an elemental milk such as Neocate). UTIs are a recognised cause of GOR and should be looked for.

Ref: M Thomson Chapter 7. In: *Baillière's Clinical Gastroenterology*. 1997;11(3):547-72.

QUESTION 9

A. FALSE   B. TRUE   C. FALSE   D. TRUE   E. FALSE

Red cell aplasia occurs in Blackfan-Diamond syndrome. Metaphyseal not epiphyseal dysostosis occurs. Average life expectancy is about 35 years and treatment with GCSF or bone marrow transplant may increase this.

QUESTION 10

A. FALSE   B. TRUE   C. TRUE   D. TRUE   E. FALSE

Bleeding is almost universally painless when occurring with a polyp. CHRPE (congenital hypertrophy of the retinal pigment epithelium) is an association with the APC (adenomatous polyposis coli) gene in 58-75% of cases and may be used in risk assessment. Peutz-Jegher's does not lead to GI tumours but does lead to malignant tumours outside the GI tract in up to 50% of cases. Pseudopolyps and inflammatory polyps in the healing phase of UC are well recognised.

QUESTION 11

A. TRUE   B. FALSE   C. FALSE   D. TRUE   E. FALSE

Oral ulceration is present in 98% of those with Behçet's disease. Recurrent aphthous ulceration is of idiopathic aetiology mainly. Perioral and perianal lesions occur in acrodermatitis enteropathica associated with a low zinc level.

Ref: Rule D, Speight P. Chapter 24. In: *Pediatric Gastrointestinal Disease*. Ed Walker A et al. St Louis. 1996.

QUESTION 12

A. TRUE   B. FALSE   C. TRUE   D. FALSE   E. TRUE

Renal blood flow is low at birth and gradually increases to adult levels (1200 ml/min or 25% of cardiac output). GFR reaches adult levels by about 1 year of age.

QUESTION   13

A. FALSE   B. TRUE   C. FALSE   D. TRUE   E. FALSE

Ileostomy and Crohn's disease related renal calculi will consist of calcium oxalate (these also occur in Type I and Type II hyperoxaluria). Cystinuria, NOT cystinosis, will cause renal calculi. Calculi from xanthinuria are radiolucent. Nephrocalcinosis is secondary to proximal RTA, and calculi to distal RTA.

QUESTION   14

A. TRUE   B. FALSE   C. FALSE   D. TRUE   E. FALSE

It is the atypical HSP which is familial, has recurrent episodes and a worse prognosis, and can present under 1 year of age. Hyperkalaemia and hypertension secondary to acute renal failure are the main causes of death. Thrombocytopaenia occurs with microangiopathic haemolytic anaemia, but coagulation defects are not usually a feature.

QUESTION   15

A. TRUE   B. FALSE   C. FALSE   D. FALSE   E. FALSE

Blood pressure and potassium levels do not distinguish. Renal failure accounts for the follwing parameters: urine osmolality < 350mosm/l; urinary sodium > 40mmol/l; urine SG < 1010; urine:plasma urea ratio < 4.1; urine:plasma osmolality ratio < 1.2; and fractional excretion of sodium >1%.

QUESTION   16

A. TRUE   B. FALSE   C. TRUE   D. TRUE   E. TRUE

Progressive liver damage due to any insult can cause cirrhosis. Alpha-1 anti-trypsin genotype is important in the pathogenesis of liver disease. Deficiency of the glycoprotein alpha-1 anti-trypsin which is a protease inhibitor correlates with genotype: PiMM is normal; PiSS has 60% activity; PiZZ has approx 15% activity of whom 20% will have neonatal cholestasis and liver involvement; and Pi null/null have no activity, but are not associated with liver disease. A Kasai porto-enterostomy must take place before 60 days of age to prevent chronic cholestatic liver disease ensuing. Liver-kidney-microsomal antibodies indicate a worse long-term prognosis in autoimmune hepatitis.

Ref: Shepherd R. Chapter 11. In: *Diseases of the liver and biliary system in childhood*. Ed Kelly D. Blackwell Science. Oxford 1999.

QUESTION   17

A. TRUE   B. TRUE   C. TRUE   D. FALSE   E. FALSE

Hepatitis A has no long-term sequelae, unlike B or C where the chance of subsequent hepatocellular carcinoma is 3-10% and 15% respectively. Hepatitis A is caused by an RNA picorna virus whereas hepatitis B is a DNA hepadna virus. Hepatitis C is caused by 6 different subtypes of an RNA virus. Types I, II and III are common in Europe and type IV in the Far East.

Ref: Davison S. Chapters 4 and 6. In: *Diseases of the liver and biliary system in childhood*. Ed Kelly D. Blackwell Science. Oxford 1999.

QUESTION 18

A. FALSE   B. FALSE   C. FALSE   D. FALSE   E. TRUE

Multisystem involvement, as is usual with mitochondrial cytopathies, especially when uncovered by fulminant liver failure with sodium valproate treatment, is a direct contraindication to liver transplant as the child will unfortunately die from irreversible neurological deterioration despite a normally-functioning liver graft. The major indication in Alagille's syndrome is poor quality of life due to intense pruritus. The host liver is virtually never left in situ as the hepatic artery and vein and portal vein are utilised for the donor organ. The chance of post-transplant CMV infection in an immunocompromised individual is highest if the donor is CMV positive, and less so if the recipient is negative.

Ref: Kelly D and Mayer D. Chapter 17. In: *Diseases of the liver and biliary system in childhood*. Ed Kelly D. Blackwell Science. Oxford 1999.

QUESTION 19

A. TRUE   B. TRUE   C. FALSE   D. FALSE   E. FALSE

LFTs will normalise within days of removal of galactose from the diet in galactosaemia. Reducing substances may be present in the urine in other infant liver disorders. Conversely galactosuria may not occur if no lactose or galactose is present in the diet. Lactate is almost always raised to above 5 mmol/l in mitochondrial cytopathies. Occasionally, choledochal cysts can be large enough to cause intestinal obstruction and bile-stained vomiting, but this does not occur in biliary atresia. Oral ursodeoxycholic acid (a synthetic bile acid inducing cholorhesis) may help in the prevention of chronic cholestasis (e.g. in cystic fibrosis or TPN-associated cholestasis), but is not helpful in the acute situation.

Ref: McKiernan P, Roberts E and Kelly D. Chapter 3. In: *Diseases of the liver and biliary system in childhood*. Ed Kelly D. Blackwell Science. Oxford 1999.

QUESTION 20

A. FALSE   B. TRUE   C. FALSE   D. FALSE   E. FALSE

The oxy-haemoglobin dissociation curve describes the relationship between the affinity of haemoglobin for oxygen and the surrounding partial pressure of oxygen.

A shift in the curve to the right (i.e. a decreased affinity of Hb for oxygen) occurs in: Acute acidosis, fever, increased pCO_2, increased 2,3 DPG and with sickle cell disease.

A shift in the curve to the left (i.e. Increased affinity for oxygen) occurs in acute alkalosis, decreased temperature, fall in pCO_2, fall in 2,3 DPG, the presence of carboxyhaemoglobin and methaemoglobin, foetal haemoglobin and with cyanotic congenital heart disease.

QUESTION 21

A. FALSE   B. FALSE   C. TRUE   D. TRUE   E. TRUE

Pyruvate kinase deficiency is autosomal recessive and is less common than G6PD deficiency. Pyruvate kinase is an enzyme involved in the Emden-Myerhof pathway, and its deficiency results in rigid RBCs. The anaemia does have relatively mild symptoms, due to a compensatory increase in 2,3 DPG levels.

The blood film shows features of haemolysis and the presence of prickle cells.

Management is with repeated blood transfusions, and splenectomy if necessary. Splenectomy can result in a massive reticulocytosis.

QUESTION   22

A. FALSE   B. FALSE   C. TRUE   D. TRUE   E. FALSE

Hereditary spherocytosis is an autosomal dominant condition and has variable expression. The defect is in the membrane protein spectrin, which results in spherical red cells, which are removed prematurely by the spleen. It is seen in Northern Europeans with an incidence of a round 1 in 5000. Neonatal jaundice occurs and may be severe, resulting in kernicterus. The condition may be asymptomatic and anaemia may not be present. Splenomegaly, leg ulcers and pigment gall stones may occur, and aplastic crises can be precipitated by parvovirus infection.

QUESTION   23

A. FALSE   B. TRUE   C. TRUE   D. FALSE   E. FALSE

von Willebrand disease is an autosomal dominant condition, however the expression is variable and it is generally more severe in females. The disorder involves low von Willebrand (vW) factor which results in reduced factor VIII activity and platelet adhesion abnormalities.

vW factor does promote platelet adhesion, and it is also a carrier protein for factor VIII.

Investigations show a prolonged bleeding time, reduced vW factor levels and reduced factor VIII activity. Platelets are of normal size.

Management of acute bleeds is with factor VIII concentrate containing vW factor. DDAVP and fibrinolytic inhibitors may also be used.

QUESTION   24

A. FALSE   B. TRUE   C. TRUE   D. TRUE   E. TRUE

Graft versus-host disease (GVHD) is due to donor T lymphocytes (not B lymphocytes) mounting an immune response to the host MHC antigens. Features of acute GVHD (within 100 days of bone marrow transplant) include cholestatic hepatitis, bloody diarrhoea and a protein-losing enteropathy. Other features of acute GVHD are a rash, fever, marrow aplasia and infections.

Active malignancy at the time of bone marrow transplantation does predispose to the disease, and there is a beneficial graft versus leukaemia (GVL) effect of the disease. T cell depletion of the donor marrow is used to prevent the disease.

QUESTION   25

A. FALSE   B. TRUE   C. FALSE   D. TRUE   E. FALSE

Brain tumours in children below 2 years of age are equally frequently supratentorial and infratentorial. Over the age of 2 years, around two thirds are posterior fossa tumours.

Medulloblastomas are usually midline posterior fossa tumours, and therefore present with truncal ataxia.

Astrocytomas are slow-growing and may be treated solely with surgical resection.

Brain stem gliomas have a poor prognosis, with a 5 year survival of around 20%.

QUESTION   26

A. TRUE   B. FALSE   C. FALSE   D. TRUE   E. TRUE

Selective IgA deficiency has a prevalence of approximately 1 in 500 in the UK and is the commonest primary immune defect. It may be asymptomatic, or result in recurrent respiratory infections or chronic diarrhoea. It is sometimes associated with IgG$_2$ and IgG$_4$ subclass deficiencies. It is also associated with autoimmune disease including SLE, Sjögren's syndrome, thyroiditis and coeliac disease. There is an increased risk of transfusion reactions in those with selective IgA deficiency.

QUESTION 27

A. FALSE   B. TRUE   C. FALSE   D. FALSE   E. TRUE

The Jak 3 mutation is seen in autosomal recessive (T-B+) SCID.

Both SCID and HIV infection may present in a similar fashion in infants with severe failure to thrive, diarrhoea and recurrent infections including opportunistic infections. X-linked agammaglobulinaemia does not present with this severe type of picture. Graft versus host features may be seen in SCID in the neonatal period. The RAG-1 and RAG-2 mutations are seen in T-B- SCID. ADA deficiency is an autosomal condition resulting from chromosome 14q13 mutation.

QUESTION 28

A. FALSE   B. FALSE   C. TRUE   D. TRUE   E. TRUE

Chediak-Higashi syndrome is an autosomal ressive condition. The immune defect is neutropenia, with neutrophil mobility and chemotaxis defects. There are giant granules in all nucleated cells. Abnormal leucocyte adhesion is seen in leucocyte adhesion defects (LAD).

Clinical features are recurrent bacterial infections and partial occulocutaneous albinism. Central and peripheral nerve lesions may occur. The EB virus can cause an accelerated phase of disease with pancytopaenia, hepatosplenomegaly and death.

QUESTION 29

A. FALSE   B. FALSE   C. FALSE   D. FALSE   E. FALSE

None of these are contraindications to vaccination.

QUESTION 30

A. TRUE   B. FALSE   C. TRUE   D. FALSE   E. TRUE

Typhoid fever causes a leucopaenia and a fever with a relative bradycardia. The illness is divided into weeks 1-4. Rose spots appear in the second week, and the third is the week of complications (e.g. seizures, perforation, pneumonia). Blood cultures are positive around 80% of the time in the first week, but this falls to 30% in the third week.

QUESTION 31

A. TRUE   B. FALSE   C. FALSE   D. TRUE   E. TRUE

Schistosoma haematobium is a trematode and causes schistosomisasis (Bilharzia). It has an intermediate host, the Bulnius snail, and penetrates human skin in the water. It then migrates to the lungs and causes Katayama fever (fever, cough, malaise, vomiting, diarrhoea, lymphadenopathy, hepatosplenomegaly). The *S. haematobium* form causes renal problems, including an increased risk of bladder cancer, and the *S. mansoni* and *S. japonicum* forms cause hepatic problems including liver fibrosis with portal hypertension.

QUESTION 32

A. FALSE   B. TRUE   C. TRUE   D. TRUE   E. TRUE

Parvovirus B19 is the cause of Fifth disease (erythema infectiosum or slapped cheek disease). It can result in a severe transient aplastic anaemia in children with haemolytic diseases such as pyruvate kinase deficiency, and is a cause of hydrops fetalis if acquired *in utero*. Sixth disease is roseola infantum (exanthem subitum), which may be caused by more than one viral agent.

QUESTION 33

A. FALSE   B. FALSE   C. TRUE   D. TRUE   E. TRUE

Homocystinuria is due to the deficiency of the enzyme cystathione synthase, resulting in accumulation of homocystine and methionine.

Clinical features include a Marfanoid habitus, fair hair and skin and blue eyes. Mental retardation is common. Lens dislocation is downwards (upwards in Marfan's syndrome). Osteoporosis and platyspondyly are seen, as are arterial and venous thromboembolism.

Management is dietary restriction of methionine with cystine supplementation (this is really only effective if started early). It may be responsive to Vitamin B_6 therapy. Betaine may be given, which allows an alternative pathway for homocystine metabolism.

QUESTION 34

A. TRUE   B. TRUE   C. FALSE   D. FALSE   E. FALSE

Hurler's disease is one of the mucopolysaccharidoses. These are lysosomal storage diseases with defective degradation and storage in the lysosomes of mucopolysaccharides (glycosaminoglycans).

Features of Hurler's disease are: coarsening of facial features, dysotosis multiplex (X-ray changes), and progressive cognitive regression. Other organs which are involved include the heart (cardiomyopathy, valve lesions), eye (corneal clouding), the skin (thickening) and the liver and spleen (hepatosplenomegaly).

They are all inherited as autosomal recessive except for Hunter's disease (X-linked recessive). Hunter's disease also involves no corneal clouding (as *hunters* need to *see* to catch their prey).

Diagnosis is by urine glycosaminoglycans (GAGS) (elevated) and specific enzyme deficiency assay on leucocytes or cultured fibroblasts. DNA analysis may also be done.

There is no specific management. Bone marrow transplantation may be suitable in some patients.

QUESTION 35

A. TRUE   B. TRUE   C. TRUE   D. FALSE   E. FALSE

Neonatal hypoglycaemia has many causes.

Polycythaemia results in hypoglycaemia due to increased glucose utilisation by RBCs. Increased utilisation is also seen in sepsis, hypothermia and birth asphyxia.

High insulin levels result in neonatal hypoglycaemia in nesidioblastosis, maternal diabetes and Beckwith-Weidemann syndrome.

Deficency of glucose substrate results in hypoglycaemia in prematurity, IUGR and some metabolic disorders. GSD 1 and 3 classically result in hypoglycaemia, but not GSD type 2.

QUESTION 36

A. FALSE B. TRUE C. TRUE D. FALSE E. FALSE

The onset of puberty in girls is usually between 8-13 years, though occurs at a younger age in the USA. The first sign is breast development, the menarche occurring most commonly at breast stage 4. The pubertal growth spurt does occur before the menarche, and at the menarche, only around 5-6 cm of further growth remains.

QUESTION 37

A. FALSE B. FALSE C. FALSE D. TRUE E. TRUE

Hyperthyroidism in children is most commonly caused by Graves' disease. It is more common in females, and it can result in advanced bone age. Graves' disease is associated with HLA B8 and idiopathic thrombocytopaenic purpura (ITP).

QUESTION 38

A. TRUE B. FALSE C. TRUE D. FALSE E. TRUE

There are investigations that establish the diagnosis of Cushing's syndrome, and those that help find the underlying cause. The ACTH level, an adrenal scan and a high dose dexamethasone suppression test will help find the underlying cause. A urine 24 hour free cortisol and the overnight dexamethasone test just help establish the diagnosis.

QUESTION 39

A. FALSE B. FALSE C. TRUE D. FALSE E. FALSE

In SIADH the serum osmolality is low (< 280 mmol/l), the plasma bicarbonate is normal with a low chloride and low sodium. The urine sodium is inappropriately high (i.e. > 30 mmol). There may be seizures, nausea, confusion and irritability. Oedema is not seen.

QUESTION 40

A. FALSE B. TRUE C. TRUE D. FALSE E. TRUE

A complete third nerve palsy results in the eye facing 'down and out'. The eyeball is rotated laterally because there is unopposed action of the superior oblique and lateral rectus muscles and therefore there is a divergent squint. This will result in double vision. The pupil is large as the parasympathetic fibres are interrupted and the sympathetic fibres are unopposed. There may be sparing of the pupil if the parasympathetic fibres are unaffected: this classically occurs in diabetic infarction of the nerve. There is a complete ptosis due to paralysis of the levator palpebrae superioris. Both the pupillary light reflex and the acommodation reflexes are lost due to the ciliary muscle paralysis.

QUESTION 41

A. FALSE B. FALSE C. TRUE D. FALSE E. TRUE

The Moro reflex disappears at around 4-5 months and the palmar grasp at around 3-4 months. The stepping reflex usually goes at 2 months, though persistence may be a sign of cerebral palsy. The forward parachute appears at around 5-6 months and stays for life.

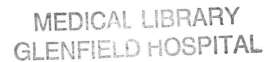

QUESTION 42

A. FALSE   B. FALSE   C. FALSE   D. FALSE   E. TRUE

Infantile spasms usually have an onset at 4-6 months. There is an identified underlying cause in the vast majority (around 80%) of cases. The EEG picture is chaotic and described as Hypsarrhythmia. There is usually but not invariably developmental regression or arrest. Vigabatrin may be used in treatment.

QUESTION 43

A. TRUE   B. TRUE   C. FALSE   D. TRUE   E. TRUE

Werdnig-Hoffmann disease is a disease of degeneration of the anterior horn cells. This results in a progressive weakness. The extra-ocular muscles are unaffected. The serum creatinine kinase (CK) is normal. Arthrogryphosis may be present due to decreased foetal movements *in utero*. Tongue fasciculation is a feature.

QUESTION 44

A. FALSE   B. FALSE   C. TRUE   D. FALSE   E. FALSE

Intussuception is most commonly seen in infants 3-9 months of age.

Henoch-Schönlein purpura is seen in infants and older children, rarely neonates.

Necrotising enterocolitis is a disease most common in neonates.

Polyps are seen in older children.

Foreign body would be seen most commonly in an older child.

QUESTION 45

A. TRUE   B. TRUE   C. FALSE   D. TRUE   E. TRUE

DNAse transforms cystic fibrosis sputum by decreasing the DNA strand size which reduces sputum viscosity. It is unhelpful in idiopathic bronchiectasis, and may even worsen lung function. It is derived from the human DNAse gene. Until 1999, clinical trials have been too short to identify a reduction in mortality or respiratory exacerbations. It is given by nebuliser.

QUESTION 46

A. TRUE   B. FALSE   C. TRUE   D. TRUE   E. TRUE

Rectal diclofenac given during surgery is used to improve post-operative pain and reduces the opiate requirement in both adults and children. Pethidine metabolites may accumulate during a sickle cell crisis and result in seizures. A very large study has demonstrated a similar incidence of gastric bleeding with ibuprofen and paracetamol.

QUESTION 47

A. TRUE   B. FALSE   C. FALSE   D. FALSE   E. FALSE

The third generation cephalosporins are β-lactamase resistant and therefore more effective against gram-negative infections unlike the first generation. Ceftazidime is the only cephalosporin with significant antipseudomonal activity. An estimated 3-7% of people with penicillin allergy cross-react with cephalosporins, and thus they are contraindicated in severe penicillin allergy. Ceftriaxone has one of the longest half-lives and thus is given only once daily.

QUESTION   48

A. TRUE   B. FALSE   C. TRUE   D. TRUE   E. TRUE

There is a higher risk of lupus erythematosis with hydralazine in slow acetylators (which represents approximately 60% of Caucasians). Sodium cromoglycate is remarkably non-toxic. Metoclopramide can cause an extrapyramidal dystonia characteristic of dopamine receptor antagonists. Ciprofloxacin can cause an arthropathy, thought the risk is small (<1.5%). Animal studies have shown an interference with immature cartilage development.

QUESTION   49

A. FALSE   B. FALSE   C. TRUE   D. FALSE   E. TRUE

The Sturge-Weber syndrome involves a facial port-wine stain roughly in the distribution of the ophthalmic and maxillary (V1 and V2) branches of the trigeminal nerve and a leptomeningeal angioma on the same side of the head causing seizures and/or hemiparesis and/or mental retardation. Glaucoma of the ipsilateral eye may be present, but is not always the case. The seizures are often refractory to treatment and surgery may be required to control them. Investigations include an MRI brain scan with gadollinium enhancement to outline the vascular anomaly. CT brain and skull X-ray may show intracranial calcification with a 'rail-road track' appearance.

QUESTION   50

A. FALSE   B. TRUE   C. FALSE   D. TRUE   E. FALSE

Pauciarticular onset JCA includes involvement of 4 or less large joints within the first 6 months of disease.

Type I disease is typically seen in females under 4 years old with knee, ankle and elbow involvement initially. Around 30% will also suffer iridocyclitis, and therefore regular slit-lamp examination is important. 20% will develop severe, extended disease. These children are ANA positive (90%); DP0201 and HLA-DR5 and 8 are associated. RhF and HLA-B27 are negative.

Type II disease is known as juvenile onset spondyloarthropathy. This is typically seen in males over 9 years old, with a lower limb arthritis, sacroiliac pain and axial disease. Acute iridocyclitis occurs in around 10%. HLA-B27 is associated in around 75% of cases, and RhF and ANA are negative.

QUESTION   51

A. TRUE   B. FALSE   C. TRUE   D. TRUE   E. TRUE

Infection of the joint space (infective arthritis) is most common in children under 2 years of age. It must be diagnosed and treated promptly to avoid destruction of the joint.

Features include an unwell, febrile child, with pseudoparesis of the affected limb. The joint involved is hot, red, tender and has a markedly reduced range of movement.

X-ray is helpful to eliminate trauma, but otherwise is normal initially. Joint USS is useful for hip infection in infants. Other investigations include FBC, CRP and ESR, blood culture, bone scan and aspiration of the infected joint.

Causes are multiple and include staphylococcus, streptococcus, meningococcus, gonnococcus and the Guinea worm. Haemophilus is more common in young children (though less with HiB vaccination), salmonella infection is seen in sickle cell disease, and yersinia is more common in iron overload. Other causes are *Borrelia burgdorfii* (Lyme disease), mycoplasma and fungal infections.

Management is with a prolonged course of intravenous antibiotics and joint immobilisation with later physiotherapy. Joint washout may be necessary, and is always so in hip disease.

QUESTION   52

A. FALSE   B. TRUE   C. FALSE   D. FALSE   E. TRUE

Osteogenesis imperfecta is a syndrome of fragile bones and is due to a defect in type I collagen. Type VII collagen defects occur in dystrophic epidermolysis bullosa. Wormian bones are seen on skull X-ray, and fractures, osteopaenia and bony deformities are also seen. The clinical features depend on the type, of which there are four. The inheritance is variable (autosomal dominant or recessive, or sporadic) depending on the type. Types I and IV are autosomal dominant, and types II and III are autosomal recessive or sporadic. Blue sclerae are seen in types I and II, and variable sclerae are seen in type III. Type IV have normal sclerae.

Other features include a conductive deafness and aortic regurgitation.

QUESTION   53

A. TRUE   B. FALSE   C. TRUE   D. TRUE   E. TRUE

Patau syndrome (47, XY, +13), or Trisomy 13, is a chromosomal defect. The features include:

Mid-facial defects and holoprosencephaly of variable severity with incomplete formation of the forebrain, the optic and olfactory nerves. They have severe mental retardation and seizures, often with hypsarrythymia on the EEG. Microcephaly, micophthalmia, iris colobomata and retinal dysplasia occur. Posterior scalp defects are seen. Cleft lip and palate, abnormal ears (low set, abnormal auricles), polydactyly of hands (and sometimes feet) and narrow hyperconvex nails are seen. Abnormal genitalia may be present, (cryptorchidism in males, uterine abnormalities in females). Cardiac abnormalities are present in around 80% of cases (VSD, ASD, PDA and dextrocardia being the most common).

Rocker-bottom feet are classically seen in Edward syndrome (Trisomy 18).

QUESTION   54

A. FALSE   B. FALSE   C. TRUE   D. FALSE   E. TRUE

Neural tube defects are classically seen with maternal carbamezipine and sodium valproate use.

Absent thymus is seen with maternal oral retinoid therapy.

Ebstein's anomaly is seen with maternal lithium therapy.

Maternal warfarin therapy will result in the foetal warfarin syndrome in approximately one third of cases. The critical period of exposure is between 6 and 9 weeks gestation. Later exposure may result in CNS defects secondary to cerebral haemorrhage.

The syndrome includes nasal hypoplasia, depressed nasal bridge and upper airway obstruction as an infant, skeletal malformations involving chondrodysplasia punctata epiphyseal stippling), brachydactyly, scoliosis and rhizomelia, nail hypoplasia, low birth weight, mental retardation and seizures. Microcephaly, agenesis of the corpus callosum, microphthalmia and hydrocephalus may occur.

QUESTION 55

A. FALSE   B. FALSE   C. TRUE   D. TRUE   E. FALSE

The neural plate appears at the 3rd week of development and is derived from ectoderm. It develops to form the neural tube, from which the brain and spinal cord are formed. The neural tube closes from a cranial to caudal direction, with completion of closure by the end of the fourth week. Failure of closure results in spina bifida. The spinal cord terminates at the end of the vertebral column at the 3rd month of development, and gradually shortens in proportion to the vertebral column, being level with L3 at birth. This is an important landmark to remember when performing lumbar punctures on infants. The cranial end of the neural tube becomes the brain. At 5 weeks of development, the brain is composed of the prosencephalon, mesencephalon and the rhombencephalon. The prosencephalon is made of the telencephalon, containing the primitive cerebral hemispheres, and the diencephalon from which develop the optic vesicles. The mesencephalic lumen becomes the aqueduct of Sylvius. The rhombencephalon is divided into the metencephalon and myelencephalon. The pons and cerebellum develop from the metencephalon, and the medulla develops from the myelencephalon.

QUESTION 56

A. FALSE   B. FALSE   C. FALSE   D. FALSE   E. FALSE

In a negatively skewed population the mode is greater than the mean.

The null hypothesis assumes that there is no significant difference between two populations.

The variance is the square of the standard deviation.

If an assay is specific there may be false negatives.

The t-test is used on parametric data.

QUESTION 57

A. TRUE   B. FALSE   C. FALSE   D. TRUE   E. FALSE

The triple test for Down's syndrome does include serum αFP (low in Down's), serum HCG (raised in Down's) and serum uE3 (low in Down's).

Nuchal fold thicknes is measured at around 11-14 weeks.

Amniocentesis carries a 1:100-200 risk of miscarriage.

Chorionic villous sampling may be done earlier than amniocentesis, at around 12 weeks.

Gestational age estimates by USS are only reliable prior to 20 weeks.

QUESTION 58

A. TRUE   B. TRUE   C. TRUE   D. FALSE   E. FALSE

Respiratory distress syndrome is specifically due to insufficient surfactant production. It is more likely if the lecithin:sphingomyelin ratio is low. It is more common in infants of diabetic mothers and in the second of twins. It is less common in infants with IUGR. Antenatal steroids help prevent the condition.

QUESTION 59

A. FALSE   B. TRUE   C. FALSE   D. TRUE   E. FALSE

Gastroschisis is much less common than omphalocoele. In gastroschisis there is a defect which is at the right paraumbilical area. In omphalocoele the defect is central.

Herniation of the liver is common in omphalocoele, as are associated extraintestinal abnormalities and chromosomal anomalies. Gastroschisis is much less likely to be associated with either chromosomal or extraintestinal abnormalities.

QUESTION 60

A. TRUE   B. TRUE   C. FALSE   D. FALSE   E. TRUE

Polyhydramnios may be due to maternal, foetal or idiopathic factors. Foetal causes include VACTERL association, where there are oesophageal abnormalities and therefore decreased swallowing, and myotonic dystrophy where the mechanism is also thought to be due to swallowing difficulties. Maternal diabetes can also cause polyhydramnios. Problems with decreased renal output such as Potter syndrome will cause oligohydramnios.

Exam 3: Questions

QUESTION 1

With the Eisenmenger reaction

- **A.** There is reversal of a previous left to right shunt
- **B.** It may result from an AVSD
- **C.** Flat p waves are seen on the ECG
- **D.** There is a soft P2
- **E.** The chest X-ray may be normal

QUESTION 2

Prostaglandin E$_2$ is indicated in the following

- **A.** Critical pulmonary stenosis
- **B.** Pulmonary atresia with a VSD
- **C.** Interrupted aortic arch
- **D.** Critical aortic stenosis
- **E.** Transposition of the great arteries

QUESTION 3

The following are characteristic of a dilated cardiomyopathy

- **A.** Jerky, ill-sustained carotid pulse
- **B.** Myocardial disarray found on cardiac biopsy
- **C.** An association with maternal IDDM
- **D.** Tricuspid regurgitation
- **E.** A reduced left ventricular shortening fraction

QUESTION 4

The following are correct

- **A.** Innocent murmurs are heard in about 30% of children
- **B.** The commonest congenital heart lesion is an ASD
- **C.** Situs solitus with dextrocardia is associated with severe congenital heart disease
- **D.** The incidence of congenital heart disease is 5 per 1000 live births
- **E.** The recurrence risk of congenital heart disease is 10% if two children are affected

QUESTION 5

The following are true

A. The foetus has its maximum number of airways at 16 weeks gestation
B. 75% of total alveoli are present at birth
C. The apex of the lung is better ventilated than the base of the lung in infants
D. The mean paO$_2$ at one week of life is two-thirds that at 5 years of age
E. Cyanosis will develop at a paO$_2$ of below 7kPa

QUESTION 6

The following are causes of localised pulmonary fibrosis

A. Bleomicin
B. Neurofibromatosis
C. Sarcoidosis
D. Langerhans cell histiocytosis
E. Post-pneumonia infection

QUESTION 7

Regarding asthma

A. Bronchodilatation with a β$_2$ agonist given by a metered-dose inhaler and spacer has been shown to be superior to doses via a nebuliser
B. The optimal particle size of aerosols for maximal lung deposition is 15-20μm
C. Electrostatic charge on the inside of a clear plastic new spacer device reduces the drug availability by about 25%
D. In pre-school children, crying increases tidal volume and also lung deposition of an aerosol
E. Only 20% of the aerosol from a nebuliser in the 6-18 year age group is deposited in the lungs

QUESTION 8

In the treatment of gastro-oesophageal reflux

A. Cisapride may cause cardiac arrhythmias only if given with macrolide antibiotics or azole antifungals
B. Omeprazole's action is on the H$_1$ receptors on oxyntic cells
C. A Nissen fundoplication involves a 75% wrap of the gastric fundus around the distal oesophagus
D. Positioning the infant prone at a 30° head-up angle is the most desirable
E. Removal of dairy produce from the diet of a breast feeding mother will not be helpful

QUESTION 9

The following is true of an osmotic diarrhoea

- **A.** Faecal sodium will be >50 mEq/l
- **B.** It may be the consequence of a transport mechanism disorder
- **C.** Bile salt/fatty acid malabsorption may be a cause of osmotic diarrhoea
- **D.** It stops when feeding is discontinued
- **E.** It may occur in Crohn's disease

QUESTION 10

Crohn's disease is more likely than ulcerative colitis if

- **A.** There is rectal sparing
- **B.** An anal tag is present
- **C.** Non-specific gastritis is seen on upper endoscopy
- **D.** Strictures are seen in the transverse colon
- **E.** Fever, malaise and lethargy are present

QUESTION 11

Acute pancreatitis in childhood

- **A.** May be caused by the use of total parenteral nutrition
- **B.** Can cause a right pleural effusion
- **C.** Is associated with Kawasaki's disease
- **D.** Causes hypercalcaemia
- **E.** Occurs in myasthenia gravis

QUESTION 12

The following are usually inherited in an autosomal fashion

- **A.** Nephrogenic diabetes insipidus
- **B.** Cystinosis
- **C.** Alport's syndrome
- **D.** Hypophosphataemic rickets
- **E.** Infantile polycystic kidney disease

QUESTION 13

In nephrotic syndrome

- **A.** A bleeding tendency occurs
- **B.** Relapse occurs in 20-30%
- **C.** Salt-poor 20% albumin is preferable to 4.5% albumin in the correction of hypoalbuminaemia
- **D.** Anti-thrombin III is increased
- **E.** Hepatitis Bs Ab is present in a proportion of cases

QUESTION 14

In an infant or child with renal vein thrombosis

A. Perinatal asphyxia is a recognised aetiological factor
B. Fibrinolytic agents have no place when it is bilateral
C. Cerebral involvement requiring prostacyclin infusion may be required
D. Which is unilateral, thrombocytopaenia is seen
E. Which is unilateral, there is associated polyuria

QUESTION 15

In a 6 year old child with a diastolic blood pressure >100 mmHg on two occasions

A. A renal cause is the most likely
B. Sublingual nifedipine is the initial treatment of choice
C. If nifedipine is ineffective then the next line of therapy is intravenous hydrallazine
D. Conn's syndrome and Cushing's syndrome may both be causes
E. And altered conscious state, Riley-Day dysautonomia is a cause

QUESTION 16

The following are true of jaundice occurring in the first month of life in term infants

A. Physiological jaundice occurs in only 20% of infants and usually lasts until the fourth week of life
B. Jaundice occurring with hypothyroidism can be conjugated or unconjugated
C. Breast feeding should be discontinued if this is determined to be the cause of jaundice after 14 days of age
D. ABO incompatability is a more common cause of severe jaundice occurring on day 1 than Rhesus incompatability
E. On fractionation of the total bilirubin, a conjugated element greater than 5% is considered pathological

QUESTION 17

Infants of hepatitis B carrier mothers

A. Should all receive hepatitis B immunoglobulin within 12 hours of birth irrespective of the mother's serology
B. Should all receive hepatitis B vaccine within 12 hours of birth irrespective of the mother's serology
C. Are more likely to acquire hepatitis B than infants of mothers with hepatitis C are to acquire hepatitis C
D. Will be unable to work in the food production industry
E. Are at greater risk of developing nephrotic syndrome if hepatitis Bs Ag positive

QUESTION 18

Hepatic glycogen storage disorders

A. Display autosomal recessive inheritance
B. Characteristically show a low cholesterol and raised triglycerides
C. Cause hepatosplenomegaly from birth
D. Frequently cause cataracts
E. Management consists of bone marrow transplantation, with or without liver transplantation

QUESTION 19

Causes of cirrhosis in childhood include

A. Phenylketonuria
B. Haemochromatosis
C. Niemann-Pick disease
D. Cystic fibrosis
E. Kwashiorkor

QUESTION 20

Regarding erythropoesis

A. Haem synthesis occurs in the mitochondria
B. Vitamin B_6 is a coenzyme involved in haem synthesis
C. The liver and spleen are the primary sites of haemopoesis during foetal life between 2-7 months
D. Erythropoietin synthesis is stimulated by high oxygen tension in the kidneys
E. Recombinant erythropoeitin may cause hypertension

QUESTION 21

In Fanconi anaemia

A. Inheritance is X-linked recessive
B. Life-expectancy is normal with androgen therapy
C. Café-au-lait patches are a feature
D. Mental retardation is common
E. Acute myeloid leukaemia often develops

QUESTION 22

In HbH disease

A. There is a deletion of 4 α-globulin genes
B. Hydrops foetalis is the usual outcome
C. Splenomegaly does not occur
D. Patients usually develop iron overload
E. Bone marrow transplant is the definitive treatment

QUESTION 23

Splenectomy

A. Results in Howell-Jolly bodies on the blood film
B. Results in an immediate marked thrombocytosis
C. Will result in susceptibility to encapsulated organisms
D. Should be avoided if possible in children under 6 years
E. Will necessitate prophylactic trimethroprim requirement for life

QUESTION 24

Neuroblastoma

A. Is a tumour arising from the neural crest cells in the parasympathetic nervous system
B. May present with cord compression
C. Arises from the adrenal medulla in 20% of cases
D. May spontaneously regress in infants
E. Associated with a chromosome 1p partial deletion, carries a better prognosis

QUESTION 25

Hodgkin's disease

A. Is a malignancy originating from histiocytes
B. Is commoner in females than males
C. Nodular sclerosing type has a good prognosis
D. Chemotherapy is indicated for Stage IA disease
E. Has a bimodal age distribution

QUESTION 26

The following have been associated with HLA-B8

A. Behçet's syndrome
B. Goodpasture's syndrome
C. Membranous glomerulonephritis
D. Dermatitis herpetiformis
E. Non-insulin dependent diabetes mellitus

QUESTION 27

In the Wiskott-Aldrich syndrome

A. Females and males are equally affected
B. There is decreased IgM
C. Mutations in the WASp gene are seen
D. There are large platelets
E. Juvenile chronic arthritis is associated

QUESTION   28

In hereditary angio-oedema

  A. Acute attacks typically involve pruritis and oedema
  B. Infection may precipitate acute attacks
  C. Antihistamine is used to prevent attacks
  D. C_2 levels are elevated in acute attacks
  E. C_1 esterase inhibitor levels are always reduced

QUESTION   29

Chicken pox

  A. Is infectious one week before the rash appearing and 2 weeks after
  B. Is an RNA virus
  C. Has an incubation period of one week
  D. Often causes pneumonia in children
  E. If acquired transplacentally can result in severe congenital malformations

QUESTION   30

Regarding syphilis

  A. Syphilis during pregnancy has a low transmission rate
  B. The secondary stage is not infectious
  C. Congenital nephrotic syndrome is a feature of congenital syphilis
  D. Epstein Barr virus infection can result in a false positive VDRL test
  E. The VDRL test remains positive for life

QUESTION   31

The following organisms and vectors are linked

  A. *Leishmania donovani* – Tsetse fly
  B. *Coccidioides immitis* – Ixodid ticks
  C. Trypanosomiasis – Sandfly
  D. Rickettsiae – Rat flea
  E. *Borellia burgdorfii* – Mosquito

QUESTION   32

Epstein–Barr virus

  A. Is a paramyxovirus
  B. Commonly results in asymptomatic infection in young children
  C. Causes a non-tender splenomegaly
  D. May cause a peripheral neuropathy
  E. Is reliably diagnosed by the Monospot test in infants

QUESTION 33

Regarding the organic acidaemias

A. They often present in the first few days of life with acidosis, vomiting and neurological features
B. They are diagnosed initially by the urinary amino acid profile
C. Acute attacks may be triggered by stress
D. Long-term management includes avoidance of catabolic states
E. They include OTC deficiency

QUESTION 34

Acute intermittent porphyria

A. Is an erythropoetic porphyria
B. Has a female preponderance
C. Is more common before puberty
D. May be precipitated by barbiturates
E. Is autosomal recessive

QUESTION 35

The following features may be suggestive of a metabolic disorder in a neonate

A. Seizures
B. Hypoglycaemia
C. Poor feeding
D. Unusual odour
E. Hyperammonaemia

QUESTION 36

Precocious puberty

A. May be caused by neurofibromatosis
B. Is more common in boys than girls
C. Is frequently pathological in boys
D. Gonadotrophin independent precocious puberty may be caused by meningitis
E. May be investigated by performing an ultrasound of the uterus

QUESTION 37

In pseudohypoparathyroidism

A. There are low levels of parathyroid hormone
B. The inheritance is autosomal recessive
C. The features include brachydactyly
D. Serum phosphate is low
E. There may be calcification of the basal ganglia

QUESTION 38

Congenital adrenal hyperplasia

A. Is associated with increased serum 17-hydroxyprogesterone levels
B. Is most commonly caused by 11-β-hydroxylase deficiency
C. Results from a genetic defect near the HLA region on chromosome 4
D. Can be diagnosed antenatally
E. May present late with precocious puberty

QUESTION 39

Hypoglycaemia in the neonatal period may be due to

A. Nesidioblastosis
B. Intrauterine growth retardation
C. Maple syrup urine disease
D. Maternal diabetes mellitus
E. Septicaemia

QUESTION 40

Regarding congenital cataracts

A. They are associated with Turner syndrome
B. They may be inherited in an autosomal dominant fashion
C. An 'oil drop' cataract is classically associated with congenital rubella syndrome
D. Those associated with prematurity may resolve spontaneously
E. They are seen with hypocalcaemia

QUESTION 41

In Apert syndrome

A. The most common presentation is with asymptomatic microscopic haematuria
B. Raised intracranial pressure is a complication
C. Mental retardation is often present
D. Mutations in the FGFR2 gene cause the syndrome
E. Syndactyly of both the fingers and toes is seen

QUESTION 42

In neurofibromatosis type 1

A. Lisch nodules are seen in the cerebral ventricles
B. More than 4 café-au-lait patches, each larger than 6 mm are needed for the diagnosis
C. Bilateral acoustic neuromas are seen
D. Renal artery stenosis may be seen
E. The gene defect is on chromsome 22q

QUESTION   43

Paralytic poliomyelitis

A. Occurs in 10% of cases of infection with poliovirus
B. Results in a symmetrical paralysis
C. Affects the upper limbs more than the lower limbs in younger children
D. Is more likely to occur in males than females
E. May rarely affect the sensory nerves

QUESTION   44

Regarding cryptorchidism

A. This is normal in 10% of males at birth
B. The testes descend through the inguinal canal in the second trimester of pregnancy
C. There is an increased risk of testicular tumour associated with cryptorchidism even after surgical correction.
D. It is seen in testicular feminisation syndrome
E. Surgical correction improves fertility

QUESTION   45

The following concerning cyclosporin are true

A. It acts by inhibiting lymphocyte replication and IL-2
B. Food and bile rarely affect absorption
C. Erythromycin increases blood levels
D. Live vaccines can be given concurrently
E. Hypertrichosis is a common side-effect

QUESTION   46

Warfarin

A. Has its peak effect 12-24 hours after starting treatment
B. Can have its effect increased by frusemide
C. May have its effect decreased by carbemazepine
D. Requires a moderation of intake of green vegetables when taken
E. Has rapid and complete absorption via the oral route

QUESTION   47

Prednisolone

A. Has little mineralocorticoid activity
B. Given orally has a slower onset of action than intravenous hydrocortisone
C. Binds to specific cell surface receptors
D. Inhibits phospholipase A_2
E. Is metabolised to prednisone

QUESTION   48

Fluconazole

A. Is fungistatic
B. Is better than nystatin in treating oropharyngeal candidiasis
C. Can cause hepatitis
D. May increase serum levels of zidvudine
E. Is not used for renal candidiasis

QUESTION   49

The EEC Syndrome (Ectrodactyly-Ectodermal Dysplasia-Clefting Syndrome)

A. Is an autosomal recessive condition
B. May include "lobster claw" hand deformity
C. May include cleft lip +/- palate
D. May include lacrimal duct stenosis
E. Is associated with intrauterine warfarin exposure

QUESTION   50

Polyarticular-onset JCA

A. Is commonly associated with iridocyclitis
B. ANA is always negative
C. Is more common in males
D. May result in micrognathia
E. RhF positive disease is seen more commonly in children under 8 years

QUESTION   51

The following are true of neonatal lupus

A. The mother usually has clinical features of SLE
B. The mother always has demonstrable anti-SSB (La) antibodies
C. Congenital heart block is reversible
D. Congenital heart block always requires treatment with insertion of neonatal pacemaker
E. The skin and blood features are transient

QUESTION   52

In osteopetrosis

A. Skeletal density is decreased
B. Blindness may be a feature
C. Splenomegaly may be seen
D. Inheritance is autosomal dominant
E. Cranial nerve palsies are a complication

QUESTION 53

The following are true of basic human cell biology

A. Somatic cells contain 23 pairs of autosomes

B. Cytosine always pairs with thiamine

C. A nucleotide is composed of one base, one deoxyribose and one phosphate group

D. A codon codes for one amino acid

E. Along a gene the 5′ direction is upstream

QUESTION 54

The following cancers are caused by the corresponding inherited mutation in the tumour suppressor gene

A. RBI gene mutation –Wilms tumour

B. AT gene mutation – Retinoblastoma

C. APC gene mutation – Familial adenomatous polyposis coli

D. WTI gene – Cowden disease (breast tumours and thyroid cancer)

E. Abl gene – Acute Lymphocytic Leukaemia (ALL)

QUESTION 55

The following result from abnormalities of development of the truncus and conus

A. Ostium primum atrial septal defect

B. Atrioventricular septal defect (AVSD)

C. Membranous ventricular septal defect

D. Tetralogy of Fallot

E. Transposition of the great arteries

QUESTION 56

The following are correct

A. A type I error is a failure to detect a significant difference when one exists

B. If the p value is >0.001 it means that the result is highly significant

C. If r is –1 there is no significant correlation between the variables

D. A sensitive test is one with very few false negatives

E. The standard deviation is greater than the standard error of the mean

QUESTION 57

The Guthrie test screens for

A. Phenylketonuria

B. Homocystinuria

C. Tyrosinaemia

D. Haemorrhagic disease of the newborn

E. Maple syrup urine disease

QUESTION   58

In congenital diaphragmatic hernia

   A. The incidence is around 1:500
   B. It is more common on the right side
   C. It may be complicated by pulmonary hypertension
   D. Resuscitation is essential prior to surgical intervention
   E. The major cause of death and morbidity is due to pulmonary hypoplasia

QUESTION   59

The following may cause neonatal thrombocytopaenia

   A. Maternal SLE
   B. Maternal idiopathic thrombocytopaenic purpura (ITP)
   C. Haemiangioma
   D. Fanconi anaemia
   E. Sepsis

QUESTION   60

Nitric oxide

   A. Is manufactured in the liver
   B. Decreases cGMP levels
   C. May result in methaemoglobinaemia
   D. Inhibits platelet function
   E. Has a half life of minutes

Exam 3: Answers

QUESTION 1

A. TRUE   B. TRUE   C. FALSE   D. FALSE   E. TRUE

The Eisenmenger reaction occurs when increased pulmonary blood flow from a left to right shunt results in increased pulmonary artery vascular resistance, pulmonary hypertension and eventually a reversal of the shunt. This is becoming less common as congenital heart disease is detected and treated earlier.

It may result from a VSD, AVSD, PDA, ASD (rarely) and any other condition with a communication between the pulmonary artery and the aorta.

The child becomes progressively dyspnoeic and cyanosed. There is a right ventricular heave and a loud P2 (due to pulmonary hypertension).

The ECG reflects these changes with right ventricular hypertrophy and tall spiked p waves. CXR shows cardiomegaly with a prominent pulmonary artery and tapering of the pulmonary vessels, but it may be normal.

QUESTION 2

A. TRUE   B. TRUE   C. TRUE   D. TRUE   E. TRUE

Prostaglandin E_2 keeps the ductus arteriosus open, and therefore is indicated with duct dependant circulations as an emergency measure.

Critical pulmonary stenosis, pulmonary atresia with a VSD and transposition of the great arteries all have duct dependant pulmonary flow.

Interrupted aortic arch and critical aortic stenosis have a duct-dependent systemic blood flow.

QUESTION 3

A. FALSE   B. FALSE   C. FALSE   D. TRUE   E. TRUE

Dilated cardiomyopathy is characterised by ventricular dilatation and impairment of function.

The features are those of cardiac failure, with arrhythmias and embolism occurring. Echocardiogram shows a poorly contracting heart with ventricular dilatation and a reduced left ventricular shortening fraction. Mitral and tricuspid regurgitation may be present.

Cardiac biopsy, if done, shows fibrosis and cells with large bizarre nuclei and white cell infiltration.

A jerky, ill-sustained arterial pulse is seen in hypertrophic obstructive cardiomyopathy (HOCM). HOCM is also associated with maternal IDDM, and on the cardiac biopsy, myocardial disarray is seen.

QUESTION 4

A. TRUE B. FALSE C. TRUE D. FALSE E. TRUE

Innocent murmurs are heard in about 30% of children.

The commonest congenital heart lesion is a VSD (30% of CHD).

Severe congenital heart disease is associated with situs solitus plus dextrocardia. And with situs inversus plus levocardia.

The incidence of congenital heart disease is 8 in 1000. The recurrence risk is 3% if one child is affected, 10% if two children are affected and 25% if three children are affected.

QUESTION 5

A. TRUE B. FALSE C. TRUE D. TRUE E. FALSE

The airways develop initially in a linear fashion. Terminal airways develop into alveoli. At birth, less than 20% of the eventual adult number of alveoli are present. The lower lung (base) is relatively collapsed in comparison to the apex in infants, and needs higher pressures to inflate - this is in contrast to adults where the base of the lung is better ventilated.

The PaO_2 at one week of age is 9 kPa, at ten weeks it is 10 kPa and at 5 years it is 13 kPa.

Cyanosis develops when there is a sufficiently high deoxyhaemoglobin concentration in the blood (3 g/dl centrally, or 5-6 g/dl peripherally). Thus an anaemic infant is less likely to develop cyanosis.

QUESTION 6

A. FALSE B. FALSE C. TRUE D. FALSE E. TRUE

Localised pulmonary fibrosis is seen in sarcoidosis, TB, systemic sclerosis and post-pneumonia infection. Bleomicin therapy, neurofibromatosis and Langerhans cell histiocytosis produce widespread pulmonary fibrosis.

QUESTION 7

A. TRUE B. FALSE C. FALSE D. FALSE E. FALSE

A metered-dose inhaler with a spacer device has been demonstrated to deliver more effectively to the lungs than a nebuliser when a good technique is employed.

The optimal particle size for aerosol deposition is 1-5 μm to allow passage into the smaller airways. In a new plastic spacer device, airway delivery is reduced by up to 85-90%. Crying may increase the tidal volume but it frequently reduces lung deposition due to closure of the vocal cords during inspiration during crying.

In the 6-18 year age group, only about 3% of the aerosol from a nebuliser is delivered to the lungs (this is doubled if a mouthpiece is used).

QUESTION 8

A. TRUE B. FALSE C. FALSE D. FALSE E. FALSE

Cardiac dysrhythmias have not been reported with cisapride alone in children at a recommended dose of 0.2 mg/kg four times daily. Omeprazole (licensed down to 2 years of age) affects the proton pump in the parietal cell by binding irreversibly to it. A Thal fundoplication is a 75% wrap around whereas a Nissen is a total wraparound. The left lateral position decreases GOR, but prone is contraindicated due to SIDS association. It is clear that small amounts of cow's milk protein passing through the breast milk are sufficient to cause vomiting due to an allergy or intolerance to cow's milk.

Ref: M Thomson. Chapter 7. In: *Baillière's Clinical Gastroenterology*. 1997:11(3):547-72.

QUESTION 9

A. FALSE   B. TRUE   C. FALSE   D. TRUE   E. TRUE

Faecal sodium will be > 90 mEq/l in a secretory diarrhoea and < 50 mEq/l in an osmotic diarrhoea. Glucose-galactose deficiency is an example of a transport mechanism disorder which may cause an osmotic diarrhoea. A secretory diarrhoea is the result of a bile salt/fatty acid malabsorption.

QUESTION 10

A. TRUE   B. TRUE   C. FALSE   D. FALSE   E. FALSE

Non-specific gastritis can occur in ulcerative colitis as well as Crohn's disease. Colonic strictures can occur in both conditions. Non-specific symptoms occur in both, although malnutrition can have a slightly increased prevalence in Crohn's disease, and UC is the more likely diagnosis if PR bleeding is present.

Ref: Leichtner A, Jackson W, Grand R. Chapter 27. In: *Pediatric Gastrointestinal Disease*. Ed Walker A. Mosby, St Louis. 1996.

QUESTION 11

A. TRUE   B. FALSE   C. TRUE   D. FALSE   E. FALSE

A left pleural effusion occurs more often than on the right. Hypocalcaemia is common.

Ref: Sidwell RU, Thomson M. *Concise Paediatrics*. Greenwich Medical Media Ltd. 2000.

QUESTION 12

A. FALSE   B. TRUE   C. FALSE   D. FALSE   E. TRUE

Nephrogenic diabetes insipidus: X-linked recessive. Cystinosis: autosomal recessive. Alport's syndrome: X-linked dominant. Hypophosphataemic rickets: X-linked dominant. Infantile polycystic kidney disease: autosomal recessive.

QUESTION 13

A. FALSE   B. FALSE   C. FALSE   D. FALSE   E. FALSE

Children are hypercoagulable in nephrotic syndrome. Relapse will occur frequently in one third, infrequently in one third and will not occur in one third. Rapid fluid shifts will occur with 20% albumin and should therefore be avoided in preference to 4.5%. Anti-thrombin III is decreased as are complement factors C_3 and C_4. Hypertriglyceridaemia and hypercholesterolaemia occur. Hepatitis B surface antigen, not antibody, is seen in some cases.

QUESTION   14

A. TRUE   B. FALSE   C. FALSE   D. TRUE   E. FALSE

Heparin, urokinase and tissue plasminogen activator have a use in the bilateral situation, as has thrombectomy. Unilateral RVT can be treated by supportive therapy with fluids, electrolyte management and treatment of any infection. HSP may cause cerebral involvement, but not RVT. USS to check IVC extension and renal enlargement is useful. The kidney becomes atrophic and should be removed if hypertension develops or repeated UTIs develop.

QUESTION   15

A. TRUE   B. FALSE   C. FALSE   D. TRUE   E. TRUE

Oral nifedipine is preferable to the sublingual route because of the potential for precipitous fall in blood pressure and hence cerebral perfusion. Similarly a labetalol infusion is preferable to hydrallazine (unless given very slowly) because hydrallazine will cause a rapid reduction in BP and hence cerebral blood flow, with the potential for causing strokes.

QUESTION   16

A. FALSE   B. TRUE   C. FALSE   D. TRUE   E. FALSE

Physiological jaundice occurs in up to 65% of term and 80% of preterm infants, and only usually lasts to day 5-7 of life. Breast milk jaundice is a diagnosis of exclusion and can last for the first 4 weeks of life, is unconjugated, poorly understood and does not require cessation of breastfeeding as it very rarely causes any pathology. Hydration and adequate milk production should be ascertained. In Rhesus disease the mother will be Rhesus negative and the baby Rhesus positive, the mother having Rhesus antibody secondary to a previous exposure. This is less common than ABO incompatability when there are maternal antibodies to A or B antigens (the mother being group O usually), and the baby being group A or B. If the conjugated element of the total bilirubin is greater than 20%, then pathology must be sought - especially if the infant is 14 days or older where biliary atresia must be excluded as early as possible.

Ref: Roberts E. Chapter 2. In: *Diseases of the liver and biliary system in childhood*. Ed Kelly D. Blackwell Science. Oxford 1999.

QUESTION   17

A. FALSE   B. TRUE   C. TRUE   D. FALSE   E. FALSE

Infants born to HBsAg +ve/HBeAb +ve mothers should receive 0.5 ml (10 mcg) i.m. vaccine within 12 hours of birth. Those born to HBsAg +ve/HBeAg +ve should also receive 200 IU i.m. hepatitis B immunoglobulin into the opposite thigh at the same time. Both groups should have a repeat vaccine dose at 1 and 6 months (in the UK). There are no exclusions to working in the food industry if the child seroconverts (in the UK). There are no predispositions to renal disease.

Ref: Davison S. Chapter 6. In: *Diseases of the liver and biliary system in childhood*. Ed Kelly D. Blackwell Science. Oxford 1999.

QUESTION   18

A. TRUE   B. FALSE   C. FALSE   D. FALSE   E. FALSE

Characteristically, cholesterol is raised > 6 mmol/l, triglycerides > 3 mmol/l, uric acid is raised > 350 μmol/l, lactate > 5 mmol/l, aminotransferases may be mildly elevated, fasting blood glucose is low < 2.5 mmol/l, but bilirubin, albumin and coagulation are normal. Cataracts occur in mucopolysaccharidoses. Lipid storage disorders cause both liver and spleen to be enlarged, but glycogen storage disorders affect the liver only. Nephromegaly may occur in Type Ia. Liver transplant may be required in Types III and IV, and rarely for Type Ia if symptomatic multiple hepatic adenomas occur, or to prevent hepatocellular carcinoma. Bone marrow transplant is useful for some lipid storage disorders but not glycogen storage disorders.

Ref: Green A and Kelly D. Chapter 9. In: *Diseases of the liver and biliary system in children*. Ed D Kelly. Blackwell Science Oxford 1999.

QUESTION 19

A. FALSE B. TRUE C. FALSE D. TRUE E. FALSE

Cirrhosis with haemochromatosis may occur as young as 7 years: 50% will have it by 11 years and all by 16 years. The lipid storage disorder Niemann-Pick disease is an abnormality of the enzyme sphingomyelinase and this can be helped by liver transplantation in Type B, but cirrhosis does not occur.

Ref: Green K and Kelly D. Chapter 9. In : Diseases of the liver and biliary system in childhood. Ed Kelly D. Blackwell Science. Oxford 1999.

Ref: Mowat A Chapter 15. In: *Liver disorders in childhood*. Butterworth-Heinemann. Oxford 1994.

QUESTION 20

A. TRUE B. TRUE C. TRUE D. FALSE E. TRUE

Haemoglobin synthesis is regulated by erythropoeitin. A low oxygen tension in the kidneys will stimulate erythropoeitin synthesis. Haemoglobin is made up of 4 polypeptide chains each containing a haem group. The haem molecules are made in the mitochondria. Vitamin B_6 (pyridoxine) is involved as a coenzyme in haem synthesis. Haemopoesis initially occurs in the yolk sac (0-2 months fetal life), then in the liver and spleen (2-7 months foetal life). The bone marrow begins to be involved from 5 months of fetal life. Recombinant erythropoeitin is given to some patients with chronic anaemia (e.g. thalassaemia) or renal failure. The side-effects include hypertension.

QUESTION 21

A. FALSE B. FALSE C. TRUE D. FALSE E. TRUE

Fanconi anaemia is a congenital aplastic anaemia which is of autosomal recessive inheritance. Features include an aplastic anaemia, growth retardation, absent radii and thumbs, microcephaly, pelvic or horseshoe kidney, café-au-lait patches and hypopigmented areas. Mental retardation occurs but is not common.

Androgen therapy delays progression of the disease, but most will succumb from bone marrow failure or acute myeloid leukaemia before the age of 30 years without a bone marrow transplant.

QUESTION 22

A. FALSE B. FALSE C. FALSE D. FALSE E. FALSE

HbH disease is an alpha thalassaemia which occurs when 3 α-globulin genes are deleted. Deletion of all 4 genes results in hydrops foetalis with Barts Hb (g4). The blood film in HbH disease shows a microcytic hypochromic anaemia with a haemoglobin of around 7-10d/dl. Golf-ball cells are also seen (aggregates of β-globin chains). They also have splenomegaly. No treatment is usually required.

QUESTION 23

A. TRUE B. TRUE C. TRUE D. TRUE E. FALSE

Splenectomy may occur naturally (autosplenectomy, e.g. in sickle cell disease) or as a result of therapeutic removal (e.g. post-traumatic injury to the spleen).

A marked thrombocytosis occurs for 2-3 weeks, which then falls to a moderate thrombocytosis.

Susceptibility to encapsulated organisms and malaria results.

Splenectomy should be avoided in young children, as they are at particular risk of infections with pneumococcus, *Haemophilus influenzae* and *Neisseria meningitidis.*

Prophylactic penicillin is required for life post-splenectomy, and triple vaccination (pneumococcal, HiB and meningovax) should be given prior to splenectomy. Malaria prophylaxis is essential when travelling to endemic areas.

Blood film post-splenectomy shows Howell-Jolly bodies, Pappenheimer granules, target cells and irregular, contracted red cells. The platelets may be high, and there may be a moncytosis and lymphocytosis.

QUESTION 24

A. FALSE B. TRUE C. FALSE D. TRUE E. FALSE

Neuroblastoma is a tumour arising from neural crest cells, but in the sympathetic (not parasympathetic) nervous system. It may present with an abdominal mass, and metastatic disease is usually present on presentation. Cord compression with paraplegia is one of the presentations. Other features are pallor, weight loss, hepatomegaly, bone pain (limp) and periorbital bruising.

Around 50% arise in the adrenal medulla, the others arising anywhere along the sympathetic chain. The neonatal tumours of stage Ds (adrenal tumour with metastases in the skin, liver or bone marrow only) may spontaneously regress.

Chromosome 1p partial deletion may be present, but this carries a worse prognosis.

QUESTION 25

A. FALSE B. FALSE C. TRUE D. FALSE E. TRUE

Hodgkin's disease is a malignancy of lymphoid tissue, but the origin of the malignant cells is unclear. It is characterised by the presence of Reed-Sternberg cells. It is twice as frequent in males than females. The histological classification includes nodular sclerosing type, which does carry a good prognosis. Stage IA disease is managed with radiotherapy alone. The age distribution is bimodal, with a peak in the mid 20s and a later peak over 50 years.

QUESTION 26

A. FALSE B. FALSE C. TRUE D. TRUE E. FALSE

HLA-B8 has been associated with membranous glomerulonephritis, dermatitis herpetiformis, coeliac disease, Addison's disease, Graves' disease, SLE, Sjögren's syndrome, myaesthenia gravis and chronic active hepatitis.

QUESTION 27

A. FALSE   B. TRUE   C. TRUE   D. FALSE   E. TRUE

Wiskott-Aldrich syndrome is an X-linked recessive condition. There are mutations in the WASp gene, resulting in a cytoskeletal defect affecting haemopoetic stem cell derivatives. There is a progressive decrease in T cells, and IgM is decreased.

The clinical features are of severe eczema, small platelets with purpura and recurrent infections. Lymphoma may occur, and autoimmune illnesses are associated, such as JCA, haemolytic anaemia and vasculitis.

QUESTION 28

A. FALSE   B. TRUE   C. FALSE   D. FALSE   E. FALSE

Hereditary angio-oedema is a condition in which acute attacks of facial swelling occur. There may be generalised oedema, including laryngeal oedema, but there is no pruritis. Acute attacks may be precipitated by infection as well as surgery, trauma, menstruation or other stress.

Antihistamines are not used as prophylaxis. Both antihistamines and steroids are usually ineffective in treatment.

During an acute attack, both C_2 and C_4 are consumed and therefore levels are reduced. C_1 esterase inhibitor is deficient in most cases, however, in a few there is a functional defect, but normal levels.

QUESTION 29

A. FALSE   B. FALSE   C. FALSE   D. FALSE   E. TRUE

Chicken pox is infectious from 2 days prior to the rash, and until there are no new crops appearing. It is a DNA virus. The incubation period is 14-21 days.

Pneumonia is rare in children but common in adults. Transplacental infection can cause severe malformations.

QUESTION 30

A. FALSE   B. FALSE   C. TRUE   D. TRUE   E. FALSE

Syphilis during pregnancy has a very high transmission rate, dependent on the stage of infection of the mother (primary and secondary syphilis being more infective). The secondary stage of syphilis is very infectious. The VDRL test has false positives, including severe infection with Epstein Barr virus. It becomes negative with treatment and can thus be used to monitor effectiveness of therapy.

QUESTION 31

A. FALSE   B. FALSE   C. FALSE   D. TRUE   E. FALSE

The following pairings of organism and vector are correct:

- *Leishmania donovani* - Sandfly
- *Coccidioides immitis* is a fungus with no vector
- Trypanosomiasis - Tsetse fly
- Rickettsiae - Rat flea and human lice
- *Borellia burgdorfii* - Ixodid ticks on deer and sheep

QUESTION 32

A. FALSE   B. TRUE   C. FALSE   D. TRUE   E. FALSE

Epstein–Barr virus infection is commonly asymptomatic in young children. A tender splenomegaly occurs in about half of symptomatic children. Neurological symptoms rarely occur, and include peripheral and cranial nerve neuropathies and meningoencephalitis. The Monospot test has frequent false negatives in infants.

QUESTION 33

A. TRUE   B. FALSE   C. TRUE   D. TRUE   E. FALSE

The organic acidaemias are a group of metabolic disorders involving raised levels of one or more organic acids. They include Maple Syrup Urine Disease (MSUD), Methylmalonic acidaemia, Isovaleric acidaemia and Propionic acidaemia. OTC is a urea cycle defect.

They do often present in the first few days of life as an acutely unwell infant with acidosis, vomiting, hypoglycaemia and neurological features. If they survive infancy they later get intermittent attacks which are triggered by stress.

Diagnosis is by the characteristic urine organic acid profile, and then confirmation is by enzyme analysis. Initial investigations include hypoglycaemia, metabolic acidosis, ketosis and hyperammonaemia.

Acute management is correction of the acidosis, rehydration, calories and haemofiltration if necessary. Long-term management includes avoidance of catabolism and a low protein diet.

QUESTION 34

A. FALSE   B. TRUE   C. FALSE   D. TRUE   E. FALSE

The porphyrias are disorders of the enzymes involved in haem biosynthesis. Acute intermittent porphyria is an acute porphyria as the name suggests and usually present after puberty as an acute attack involving abdominal, neurological, cardiovascular and neuropsychiatric symptoms. The acute porphyrias are autosomal dominant. Attacks may be precipitated by many drugs including barbiturates, stress (illness or psychological), calorie reduction and menstruation. It is more common in females. Investigations include urine analysis (urine becomes red-brown on standing); urinary ALA and PBG are raised during attacks. Serum ALA and PBG are elevated during attacks. Stool uroporphyrin and coproporphyrin are raised.

Screening of relatives is necessary by checking erythrocyte PBG deaminase levels (decreased) and ALA synthetase levels (raised).

QUESTION 35

A. TRUE   B. TRUE   C. TRUE   D. TRUE   E. TRUE

All of these features may be seen in metabolic disorders. Often the child appears normal at birth.

Neonatal features include poor feeding, vomiting, hypoglycaemia, lethargy, seizures, irritability, coma and unusual smell. Hyperammonaemia is seen in some disorders.

Later presentation may be with failure to thrive, developmental regression, seizures, encephalopathy, and intermittent episodes of vomiting, acidosis, hypoglycaemia or coma triggered by stress.

QUESTION 36

A. TRUE   B. FALSE   C. TRUE   D. FALSE   E. FALSE

Precocious puberty may be caused by early activation of the hypothalamic-pituitary-gonadal axis (Gonadotrophin-dependent). Neurofibromatosis and meningitis may both result in this type of precocious puberty. Gonadotrophin-independent precocious puberty is not driven centrally and may be caused by, for example, adrenal tumours. Precocious puberty is much more common in girls than boys, but is mostly pathological when occuring in boys. A pelvic ultrasound looking at the ovaries, but not the uterus, would be useful in investigating the cause.

QUESTION 37

A. FALSE   B. FALSE   C. TRUE   D. FALSE   E. TRUE

Pseudohypoparathyroidism is due to an end organ resistance to parathyroid hormone (PTH), and therefore the PTH is high. The condition is inherited in an autosomal dominant fashion. The phenotype includes brachydactyly with a short 4th metacarpal, short stature, a round face and bow legs. There may be calcification of the basal ganglia, mental retardation and cataracts. Serum calcium is low, phosphate high and alkaline phosphatase high.

QUESTION 38

A. TRUE   B. FALSE   C. FALSE   D. TRUE   E. TRUE

Congenital adrenal hyperpasia is an autosomal dominant condition, and the genetic defect is near the HLA region, which is on chromosome 6 not 4. The most common type is 21-hydroxylase deficiency, and this is associated with a raised serum 17-hydroxyprogesterone level. The condition can be diagnosed antenatally. It may present with ambiguous genitalia with masculinisation of a female infant. Or it can present with an adrenal crisis at around 2-3 weeks of age. It can present later in childhood with tall stature (eventual short stature), hypertension, hirsutism, precocious puberty and advanced bone age.

QUESTION 39

A. TRUE   B. TRUE   C. TRUE   D. TRUE   E. TRUE

Hypoglycaemia in the neonatal period has many causes, and can be divided into transient and persistent hypoglycaemia.

Intrauterine growth retardation, maternal diabetes mellitus and septicaemia are causes of transient hypoglycaemia. Maple syrup urine disease and nesidioblastosis are causes of persistent hypoglycaemia.

QUESTION 40

A. TRUE   B. TRUE   C. FALSE   D. TRUE   E. TRUE

Congenital cataracts have many causes. They are seen in Turner syndrome among other inherited chromosomal disorders including trisomy 21. They may be inherited in autosomal dominant fashion. 'Oil drop' cataracts are seen in Galactosaemia. Cataracts associated with prematurity may resolve spontaneously. They are seen in metabolic disorders including hypocalcaemia and in infants of diabetic mothers.

QUESTION 41

A. FALSE   B. TRUE   C. TRUE   D. TRUE   E. TRUE

Apert syndrome is one of the craniosynostosis syndromes. It involves premature closure of multiple cranial sutures. Raised intracranial pressure is a complication and mental retardation is present in the majority of cases. Syndactyly is seen of both the fingers and toes. It is caused by mutations in the fibroblast growth factor receptor 2 gene (FGFR2). It is not to be confused with Alport syndrome, the most common type of hereditary nephritis.

QUESTION 42

A. FALSE   B. FALSE   C. FALSE   D. TRUE   E. FALSE

Neurofibromaosis type 1 (NF-1) is the most common type of neurofibromatosis. Lisch nodules are hamartomas which may be seen in the iris. One of the diagnostic criteria is more than 5 café-au-lait patches, each greater than 6 mm in diameter. Bilateral acoustic neuromas are seen in NF-2. Renal artery stenosis is an associated feature, and therefore blood pressure should be checked on follow-up of these children. The gene defect is on chromosome 17q (22q is NF-2).

QUESTION 43

A. FALSE   B. FALSE   C. FALSE   D. TRUE   E. FALSE

Paralytic poliomyelitis is a rare occurrence, and is seen in less than 1% of cases of infection with the polio virus. It results in an asymmetrical paralysis, affecting the lower limbs more commonly than the upper limbs in the younger children. It is more likely to occur in males, and there is no sensory involvement.

QUESTION 44

A. FALSE   B. FALSE   C. TRUE   D. TRUE   E. TRUE

Cryptorchidism is normal in about 3.5% of newborn males.

The testes descend in the third trimester of pregnancy.

The risk of testicular tumour remains increased after surgical correction, but it is easier to spot earlier.

Testicular feminisation syndrome results from a defective response to testosterone. There is usually cryptorchidism at birth.

Surgical correction does improve fertility.

QUESTION 45

A. TRUE   B. FALSE   C. TRUE   D. FALSE   E. TRUE

Cyclosporin acts by inhibiting lymphocyte replication (IL-2 is a T cell growth factor) and eosinophil function. Blood levels are inconsistent and they are difficult to predict because food and bile affect the absorption. Both macrolide antibiotics and imidazole antifungals inhibit the metabolism of cyclosporin and therefore increase blood levels. Live vaccines are contraindicated in immunosuppressed patients. Patients need to be warned of possible hypertrichosis, but it is not as serious a side-effect as renal deterioration which necessitates regular BP and GFR monitoring.

QUESTION 46

A. FALSE B. TRUE C. TRUE D. TRUE E. TRUE

The peak effect of warfarin occurs after 1-3 days as the existing clotting factors are depleted. Frusemide increases the effect of warfarin by displacement from albumin. Carbamazepine is a liver enzyme inducer and thus may decrease the effect of warfarin. Green vegetables contain a high content of vitamin K and thus a high intake may reduce the effectiveness of warfarin. Warfarin via the oral route has a 100% bioavailability.

QUESTION 47

A. TRUE B. FALSE C. FALSE D. TRUE E. FALSE

Both oral prednisolone and intravenous hydrocortisone have a peak onset within 1-2 hours, and oral prednisolone is rapidly absorbed. Prednisolone crosses the cell membrane and then binds to cytoplasmic receptors inducing modification of DNA transcription. Prednisolone does inhibit phospholipase A_2, and thus inhibits prostaglandins and leukotrienes. Prednisone is metabolised to prednisolone.

QUESTION 48

A. TRUE B. TRUE C. TRUE D. TRUE E. FALSE

Fluconazole is fungistatic. It interferes with cytochrome P450 causing defective cell membrane production and inability to reproduce. In a trial of 159 children with oropharyngeal candidiasis, fluconazole caused a clinical clearance in 91%, compared to only 51% when treated with nystatin. Fluconazole can affect the human cytochrome enzyme and cause a hepatitis, but it is more fungal specific than itraconazole or ketoconazole. Fluconazole is useful in renal candidiasis as in children up to 65% is excreted unchanged in the urine (this rises to about 90% in adults).

QUESTION 49

A. FALSE B. TRUE C. TRUE D. TRUE E. FALSE

The EEC syndrome is one of the ectodermal dysplasias, which are a group of disorders involving defects of nails, hair, teeth and skin.

The EEC syndrome is an autosomal dominant condition. All features are variable and they include ectodermal dysplasia (thin, dry skin, wispy hair, no eyelashes), cleft lip +- cleft palate (72%), peg-shaped teeth, lacrimal duct stenosis (84%) and ectrodactyly ('lobster claw' deformity of the hands and feet).

Other diseases in this group include hypohydrotic ectodermal dysplasia (reduced or absent sweat glands) and hydrotic ectodermal dysplasia (normal sweating).

QUESTION 50

A. FALSE B. FALSE C. FALSE D. TRUE E. FALSE

Polyarticular-onset JCA is involvement of multiple joints (4 or more joints by definition). It is more common in females.

Children under 8 years mostly have RhF negative disease, with assymetrical disease particularly involving the spine and temperomandibular joint (TMJ). Iridocyclitis is seen occasionally (in around 5%). RhF positive disease is most common in those over 8 years, and is a symmetrical disease involving particularly the hands, feet and hips.

The disease can lead to problems as a result of distorted growth. Particular problems are micrognathia due to TMJ involvement which causes problems with dental hygiene and anaesthetics. Cervical spine fusion or subluxation may occur. Hip disease can result in limb shortening and knee disease in valgus deformity.

ANA may be positive.

QUESTION 51

A. FALSE   B. FALSE   C. FALSE   D. FALSE   E. TRUE

Neonatal lupus usually occurs in infants of mothers with anti-SSA (Ro) antibodies, and many have anti-SSB (La) antibodies also. Maternal disease is not usually clinically evident. The antibodies are IgG and result in transplacentally acquired disease. Clinical features are not inevitable and are variable. They include neonatal lupus rash, and haematological manifestations (thrombocytopaenia, anaemia, leucopaenia). These features are transient, usually resolving within the first few months of life. Congenital heart block is caused by damage to the foetal conducting tissue by the maternally derived antibodies. This damage is permanent, and in around half of cases a pacemaker is required, though this is not inevitable.

Investigations include an ECG, FBC and autoantibody profile including ANA, Ro, La, anti-platelet antibodies and Coombs' test.

QUESTION 52

A. FALSE   B. TRUE   C. TRUE   D. FALSE   E. TRUE

In osteopetrosis, skeletal density is increased and the bones are brittle. It is also known as Marble Bone Disease and occurs in several forms. Clinical features include those of hyperostosis and marrow failure.

Marrow failure results in anaemia, thrombocytopaenia, susceptibility to infections and extramedullary haemopoesis (with hepatosplenomegaly).

Hyperostosis may cause optic atrophy and later blindness, deafness and cranial nerve palsies.

X-rays show increased bone density, clubbed metaphyses, osteosclerosis and a "rugby jersey" pattern of the spine.

The inheritance depends on the form.

QUESTION 53

A. FALSE   B. FALSE   C. TRUE   D. TRUE   E. TRUE

Somatic cells are diploid and contain 22 pairs of autosomes and 1 pair of sex chromosomes (i.e. 46 chromosomes altogether). Gametes contain 22 autosomes and 1 sex chromosome (i.e. 23 chromosomes altogether).

Nitrogenous bases in the DNA double helix exhibit complementary base pairing. Cytosine always pairs with guanine, and adenine always pairs with thiamine (or uracil in RNA).

A nucleotide is a unit of one base, one deoxyribose and one phosphate group.

A codon is a sequence of three bases and it codes for one amino acid via the genetic code.

The sugar-phosphate backbone has a 5' and a 3' end. The DNA strand grows from the 5' to the 3' direction, with bases added at the 3' end. The 5' direction is described as upstream and the 3' and downstream.

QUESTION 54

A. FALSE   B. FALSE   C. TRUE   D. FALSE   E. FALSE

The following are the correct associations:

- RBI gene mutations (on chromosome 13q14) – Retinoblastoma, osteosarcoma
- AT gene (chromosome 11q22) – Ataxia telangiectasia
- APC gene (chromosome 5q21) – Familial adenomatous polyposis coli
- WTI gene (chromosome 11p13) – Wilms tumour
- Abl is an oncogene, not a tumour suppressor gene, and is associated with ALL

QUESTION 55

A. FALSE   B. FALSE   C. FALSE   D. TRUE   E. TRUE

Abnormalities of development of the truncus and conus may result in Tetralogy of Fallot, transposition of the great arteries, and truncus arteriosus.

Ostium primum septal defect and AVSD result from abnormalities of development of the atrioventricular canal. Membranous ventricular septal defect results from abnormality of development of the interventricular septum.

QUESTION 56

A. FALSE   B. TRUE   C. FALSE   D. TRUE   E. TRUE

A type I error is when a difference is considered to be significant when no such difference exists. A type II error is described in the question.

A p value of 0.001 does mean that the result is highly significant.

r is Pearson's correlation coefficient. A value of –1 indicates a perfect negative relationship between the variables.

A sensitive test is one with few false negatives.

The standard deviation is greater than the standard error of the mean, as it is calculated by dividing the standard deviation by the square root of the sample size.

QUESTION 57

A. TRUE   B. TRUE   C. FALSE   D. FALSE   E. TRUE

The Guthrie test is done at the end of the first week of life and is a biochemical screen for phenylketonuria, galactosaemia, maple syrup urine disease, homocystinuria and hypothyroidism. In some parts of the country it is used to screen for cystic fibrosis and haemoglobinopathies.

QUESTION 58

A. FALSE   B. FALSE   C. TRUE   D. TRUE   E. TRUE

Congenital diaphragmatic hernia has an incidence of around 1:4000. About 80% occur on the left side (Bochdalek type). Resuscitation is necessary prior to surgical correction with nasogastric tube and aspiration, circulatory support, intubation and ventilation as necessary. The major problem is due to underdevelopment of the lungs, and pulmonary hypertension may occur.

QUESTION 59

A. TRUE   B. TRUE   C. TRUE   D. TRUE   E. TRUE

Neonatal thrombocytopaenia results from an increased destruction of platelets, or from decreased production. There are many causes and they include maternal SLE and maternal ITP. A haemangioma if giant or multiple can result in increased platelet destruction and thrombocytopaenia. Any form of sepsis can cause thrombocytopaenia. Fanconi anaemia can cause neonatal thrombocytopaenia. Other causes to consider include iatrogenic (drugs), diffuse intravascular coagulation, a large thrombosis and other congenital abnormalities (e.g. trisomy 18).

QUESTION 60

A. FALSE   B. FALSE   C. TRUE   D. TRUE   E. FALSE

Nitric oxide is used as a selective vasodilator, acting particularly on the pulmonary smooth muscle. It is a neurotransmitter manufactured by vascular endothelium and macrophages. It acts via increasing cGMP levels. Other effects include inhibition of platelet function and it may cause methaemoglobinaemia.

Exam 4: Questions

QUESTION 1

In a patient with a small VSD

A. Symptoms are usually present at birth
B. The risk of endocarditis is an indication for closure of the defect
C. The ECG is usually normal
D. If the systolic murmur is loud the prognosis is worse
E. 10% will close spontaneously in the first few years of life

QUESTION 2

The following are features of a supraventricular tachycardia

A. The tachycardia responds to adenosine
B. Fusion beats are present
C. There is AV dissociation
D. The heart rate is always regular
E. Capture beats are present

QUESTION 3

Peripheral pulmonary stenosis is seen in

A. Alagille syndrome
B. Marfan's syndrome
C. Klinefelter's syndrome
D. Congenital rubella syndrome
E. William's syndrome

QUESTION 4

A right sided aortic arch is seen with

A. Ebstein's anomaly
B. Tetralogy of Fallot
C. Congenital vascular ring
D. Pulmonary atresia
E. Truncus arteriosus

QUESTION 5

In *pneumocystis carinii* pneumonia

A. Presentation in infants is usually with acute onset of dyspnoea
B. Investigation may require bronchoalveolar lavage
C. Septrin may cause a neutropaenia
D. The chest X-ray is normal on presentation in around a quarter of cases
E. Post-infection prophylaxis with septrin is sometimes necessary in the immunompromised

QUESTION 6

Cystic adenomatoid malformation (CAM) of the lung

A. Is the most common congenital malformation of the lung
B. Rarely results in midline shift with compression of the opposite lung
C. May present with recurrent chest infections
D. Is associated with Turner's syndrome
E. Is managed with surgical resection

QUESTION 7

Regarding cystic fibrosis

A. Nasal polyps in childhood and adolesence are virtually pathognomonic of cystic fibrosis
B. It may present in infancy with severe gastro-oesophageal reflux
C. The commonest cause of a respiratory exacerbation during infancy is *Haemophilus influenzae*
D. Flucloxacillin does not interfere with the sweat test
E. Treatment of allergic bronchopulmonary aspergillosis is with itraconazole as first line therapy

QUESTION 8

In a child who appears to have malabsorption

A. Anti-endomysial antibody is 99.5% sensitive for coeliac disease
B. Faecal elastase is the most practically useful test for pancreatic insufficiency
C. Giardiasis may be diagnosed by faecal examination in 70% of cases
D. A small bowel biopsy is necessary for the diagnosis of abetalipoproteinaemia
E. Primary lactase deficiency is a common cause

QUESTION 9

Features of a non-organic origin for recurrent abdominal pain in children and adolescents are

A. Early morning wakening with pain
B. Absence of dysuria
C. Predominance in girls
D. A family history of atypical migraine
E. Negative correlation with *Helicobacter pylori* serological positivity

QUESTION   10

Recognised pathology and complications of Crohn's disease include

A. Toxic megacolon
B. Increased presence of megakaryocytes
C. Calcium oxalate renal calculi
D. Caseating granulomas
E. Eventual diminished adult height if testicular volume is 5-10 ml at 17 years of age

QUESTION   11

Regarding micronutrient and vitamin deficiencies

A. Dermatitis, dementia, and diarrhoea occurs with a deficiency of niacin (or nicotinamide)
B. Symmetrical polyneuropathy occurs with thiamine deficiency
C. Raised S-T segments on ECG can occur with vitamin A deficiency
D. Selenium deficiency occurs within 6 weeks of commencement of total parenteral nutrition and can cause pericarditis
E. Vitamin A is found mainly in fish when a child is on a dairy-free diet

QUESTION   12

Atrial naturetic peptide

A. Increases glomerular filtration rate
B. Decreases blood pressure
C. Decreases renin-angiotensin-aldosterone system action
D. Is secreted from the cardiac atria in response to increased stretch, increased pressure and increased osmolality
E. Causes peripheral vasoconstriction

QUESTION   13

Low complement levels are a finding in

A. Recurrent severe pyelonephritis
B. Mesangiocapillary glomerulonephritis
C. Post-streptococcal glomerulonephritis
D. Congenital nephrotic syndrome
E. Focal segmental glomerulonephritis

QUESTION   14

Proximal renal tubular acidosis is associated with

A. Proximal tubular bicarbonate secretion
B. Rickets
C. Aminoaciduria
D. Hypochloraemia
E. Interstitial nephritis

QUESTION   15

Renal malformations occur in the following

A. Crohn's disease
B. Ulcerative colitis with positive pANCA
C. Tuberous sclerosis
D. Hemihypertrophy
E. DiGeorge syndrome

QUESTION   16

Biliary atresia is characterised by

A. An absence of a gallbladder on fasting ultrasound
B. Biliary duct proliferation on liver biopsy
C. Poor uptake of radioisotope into the liver after pre-administration of phenobarbitone for 5 days
D. Facial dysmorphism with hypertelorism, deep-set eyes and a small mandible
E. Conjugated hyperbilirubinaemia in the first 24 hours of life

QUESTION   17

The following are true of hepatitis B

A. Interferon α may seroconvert approximately 40% of infected children
B. HBsAb indicates a carrier state
C. 5-10% of infected children will develop fulminant hepatic failure
D. Hepatitis D virus can only occur in the presence of hepatitis B virus
E. HBeAb indicates high infectivity

QUESTION   18

In children with primary hepatic tumours

A. Hepatocellular carcinoma is commoner under the age of 4 than hepatoblastoma
B. Abdominal pain will be the presenting feature in 90%
C. Jaundice occurs in less than 10%
D. Plain abdominal X-ray will demonstrate calcification in 40-50% of hepatocellular carcinomas
E. Hepatoblastoma has a well-established link with Beckwith-Weidemann syndrome and hemihypertrophy

QUESTION   19

In paracetamol-induced hepatotoxicity in childhood

A. Hypoglycaemia is the commonest presenting feature
B. Concomitant ingestion of enzyme-inducers such as anti-convulsant drugs may increase risk of hepatotoxicity
C. Treatment with N-acetyl cysteine should be delayed until paracetamol levels are known
D. Subsequent autoimmune hepatitis is commoner than in the general population
E. A Type IV systemic hypersensitivity reaction plays a part in the liver damage

QUESTION 20

The following are true regarding sideroblastic anaemia

- **A.** It occurs as an X-linked recessive disease
- **B.** It is seen in lead poisoning
- **C.** A dimorphic blood film is often present
- **D.** Pyridoxine may be used in therapy
- **E.** Ring sideroblasts are seen in the marrow

QUESTION 21

In Diamond-Blackfan syndrome

- **A.** A neutropaenia may be present
- **B.** Presentation is usually in late childhood
- **C.** Erythropoeitin levels are raised in the blood
- **D.** Triphalangeal thumbs are seen
- **E.** The blood film shows a microcytic anaemia

QUESTION 22

Regarding idiopathic thombocytopaenic purpura

- **A.** It is associated with Epstein Barr infection
- **B.** Antiplatelet IgG antibodies are seen
- **C.** It usually occurs during a viral infection
- **D.** Chronic disease occurs in about a third of cases
- **E.** Transfused platelets are quickly destroyed

QUESTION 23

Causes of splenomegaly include

- **A.** Osteopetrosis
- **B.** Christmas disease
- **C.** Diamond-Blackfan syndrome
- **D.** Brucellosis
- **E.** Neimann-Pick disease

QUESTION 24

The following are associated with Wilms tumour

- **A.** Mental retardation
- **B.** Neurofibromatosis
- **C.** Prader-Willi syndrome
- **D.** Hemiplegia
- **E.** Aniridia

QUESTION   25

The following are associated with a good prognosis in acute lymphoblastic leukaemia (ALL)

A. Male sex
B. Age below 2 years at presentation
C. Hyperdiploidy
D. Translocation 4:11
E. Initial WCC low

QUESTION   26

Regarding immunoglobulins

A. IgA is present in adult levels at birth
B. IgG levels fall in the months after birth
C. IgG is present in adult levels at birth
D. IgM reaches adult levels by puberty
E. Raised IgM levels at birth are seen in intra-uterine infection

QUESTION   27

Regarding ataxia telangiectasia

A. Cell mediated immunity is impaired
B. IgA levels are normal
C. There is a sensitivity to ionising radiation
D. There are mutations in the ATM gene
E. α-fetoprotein (AFP) is elevated

QUESTION   28

The following vaccines should be avoided in a child with a history of severe allergy to eggs

A. Diphtheria
B. MMR
C. Tetanus
D. Yellow fever
E. Influenza

QUESTION   29

In measles infection

A. The eruptive stage is infectious
B. Forchheimer spots are seen
C. The incubation period is 14–21 days
D. Koplik spots are pathognomonic
E. There are EEG abnormalities during infection in up to 50% of cases

QUESTION 30

Lyme disease

A. Is a Rickettsial infection
B. Is transmitted by sandflies
C. May be diagnosed by measuring serum antibodies
D. Is a cause of erythema marginatum
E. Causes a chronic recurrent arthritis in most cases if untreated

QUESTION 31

In Rabies

A. The virus enters at the bite wound and spreads via the lymphatics
B. There is a vaccine which is live attenuated
C. The average incubation period is less than 4 weeks
D. Aerophobia is pathognomonic
E. Dumb rabies is acquired from bats

QUESTION 32

The following are true regarding the enteroviruses

A. They may cause an acute haemorrhagic conjunctivitis
B. Coxsackie A and B are the most common causes of Ludwig's angina
C. They are the most common cause of aseptic meningitis
D. Rotavirus is one of the enteroviruses
E. The major cause of hand foot and mouth disease is Coxsackie A10

QUESTION 33

Urea cycle defects

A. Are associated with raised serum ammonia levels
B. Initial diagnosis is usually made by plasma amino acid profile and urine orotic acids.
C. Include isovaleric acidaemia
D. Are all autosomal recessive disorders
E. May present with developmental delay

QUESTION 34

Chondrodysplasia punctata is seen in

A. Conradi–Hunermann syndrome
B. Citrullinaemia
C. Zellweger syndrome
D. X-linked adrenoleucodystrophy
E. Warfarin toxicity

QUESTION 35

First line investigations in a metabolic screen include

A. Serum ammonia
B. Urine amino acids
C. Plasma amino acids
D. Enzyme analysis from fibroblast culture
E. Blood gas

QUESTION 36

Short stature may be caused by

A. Noonan syndrome
B. An XYY karyotype
C. Testicular feminisation syndrome
D. Chronic illness, if disproportionate
E. XY/XO mosaicism

QUESTION 37

In polycystic ovary syndrome

A. There may be secondary amenorrhoea
B. There is early onset osteoporosis
C. There is a raised FSH:LH ratio
D. Prolactin is moderately raised
E. The oral contaceptive pill may be used in treatment

QUESTION 38

In type I diabetes mellitus

A. First presentation in children is usually under the age of 4 years
B. Presentation is most common in winter
C. Most children have islet cell antibodies on first presentation
D. A sibling of a child with the disease has a 1 in 40 risk of developing it also
E. There is an association with HLA DR4

QUESTION 39

Infants of diabetic mothers are at risk of the following

A. Respiratory distress syndrome
B. Sacral agenesis
C. Hyperglycaemia
D. Polycythaemia
E. Hypoplastic left colon

QUESTION   40

Regarding aniridia

- **A.** Cataract is often associated
- **B.** Visual acuity is unaffected
- **C.** It may be seen with chromosome 11p deletions
- **D.** It is mostly sporadic
- **E.** All patients should be screened with regular renal ultrasound scans

QUESTION   41

Absence seizures

- **A.** Usually last less than 30 seconds
- **B.** Usually are preceded by an aura
- **C.** If typical, may involve myotonic movements
- **D.** May have a post-ictal state
- **E.** A typical 1 per second spike and wave pattern is seen on the EEG

QUESTION   42

The following may cause acute ataxia

- **A.** *Varicella* infection
- **B.** Phenytoin
- **C.** Joubert disease
- **D.** Cerebellar tumour
- **E.** Abetalipoproteinaemia

QUESTION   43

In myaesthenia gravis

- **A.** Edrophonium is used in treatment
- **B.** The external occular muscles are unaffected
- **C.** There is an association with HLA-B8, DR3
- **D.** There are IgA antibodies to acetylcholine receptors
- **E.** The baby of a mother with myaesthenia gravis may develop a transient form of the disease

QUESTION   44

Legg-Calve-Perthes disease

- **A.** Involves aseptic necrosis of the tibial tubercle
- **B.** Is 5 times more common in males than females
- **C.** Is bilateral in around half of cases
- **D.** Is generally managed conservatively in a child under 6 years
- **E.** Is one of the osteochondritides

QUESTION 45

Concerning iron poisoning

A. Activated charcoal is of proven benefit

B. Clinical improvement at a few hours will result in a better outcome

C. Pyloric stenosis is a well recognised complication

D. Severe hepatic necrosis may occur within 24 hours

E. Desferrioxamine can be given orally

QUESTION 46

Regarding anticonvulsants

A. The anti-epileptic effect of intravenous diazepam lasts 60–90 minutes

B. Phenytoin appears to reduce cognitive function more than carbemazepine or sodium valproate

C. The estimated risk of congenital malformations in women receiving phenytoin during pregnancy is around 2%

D. A transient leucopenia and thrombocytopenia occurs in up to 10% of patients on carbamazepine

E. Phenytoin is used for absence seizures

QUESTION 47

Dopamine

A. Has a half-life of 2 minutes

B. Causes release of noradrenaline from nerve endings

C. Increases renal blood flow

D. Is inactivated by acidic solutions

E. Exerts inotropic action via B_1 receptors

QUESTION 48

The following concerning vincristine are true

A. Bone marrow suppression occurs about 48 hours after treatment

B. A transient neuropathy is a recognised side-effect

C. Extravasation generally causes little problem

D. It is cell cycle specific for the M-phase

E. The dose needs increasing in biliary tract disease

QUESTION 49

Waardenberg syndrome

A. Includes deafness in 80% of cases

B. Includes vitiligo

C. Type II is caused by mutations in the PAX3 gene

D. Includes mental retardation

E. Is associated with Hirschsprung's disease

QUESTION   50

Systemic-onset juvenile chronic arthritis

- **A.** Is a clinical diagnosis of exclusion
- **B.** Classically involves a salmon-pink rash
- **C.** Amyloidosis is a late feature
- **D.** RhF is usually positive
- **E.** A polyarthritis rarely occurs

QUESTION   51

In juvenile onset dermatomyositis

- **A.** "En coup de sabre" lesion on the forehead may be seen
- **B.** There is a low mortality if untreated
- **C.** It is associated with DQA1★0501
- **D.** A heliotrope violaceous rash over the eyelids is pathognomonic
- **E.** Subcutaneous calcium deposits may be seen

QUESTION   52

Causes of blue sclerae include

- **A.** Ehlers Danlos syndrome
- **B.** Osteogenesis imperfecta Type IV
- **C.** Marble bone disease
- **D.** Pseudoxanthoma elasticum
- **E.** Phenylketonuria

QUESTION   53

The polymerase chain reaction

- **A.** Is a technique to sequence DNA
- **B.** Can be used on very long DNA sequences (i.e. several kb long)
- **C.** May be used in antenatal chorionic villous sampling
- **D.** Involves cycles of heating and cooling
- **E.** May be used on DNA in a sample of blood stain that is several years old

QUESTION   54

Diseases associated with tri-nucleotide repeat expansions include

- **A.** Friedreich's ataxia
- **B.** Miller-Dieker syndrome
- **C.** Huntington's disease
- **D.** Myotonic dystrophy
- **E.** Myoclonic epilepsy with ragged red fibres (MERRF)

QUESTION   55

The following are true of Trisomy 21

A. PDA is the commonest cardiac anomaly seen
B. Hypotonia is common in infancy
C. Risk of recurrence is 100% if a parent has the translocation 21:21
D. The genetic cause is non-disjunction in approximately 75% of cases
E. Karyotyping is essential

QUESTION   56

Regarding significance tests

A. A paired t-test is used to compare two independant samples
B. The Mann-Whitney test is used on parametric data
C. The unpaired t-test is used on non-parametric data
D. Wilcoxon is the non-parametric equivalent of the paired t-test
E. The Chi-squared test may be used on parametric or non-parametric data

QUESTION   57

In Erb's palsy

A. The injury is to the C7, C8 and T1 nerve roots of the brachial plexus
B. The arm is classically held in the 'waiter's tip' position
C. There is a wrist drop
D. All will recover fully over weeks to months
E. Physiotherapy is necessary to prevent contractures

QUESTION   58

The following are true of infants of maternal drug abusers

A. Rhinorrhea is a feature of drug withdrawal
B. Decreased sensory stimuli have a beneficial effect on the drug-withdrawing infant
C. Lacrimation is increased
D. The infants have an increased metabolic rate
E. There is an increased risk of SIDS

QUESTION   59

The following are causes of unconjugated neonatal hyperbilirubinaemia

A. Biliary atresia
B. Gilbert's disease
C. Alagille syndrome
D. Hirschsprung's disease
E. Galactosaemia

QUESTION   60

Regarding neonatal seizures

  A. They are usually terminated if the limb is held

  B. If myoclonic, they often indicate a severe brain disturbance

  C. Most neonatal seizures are obvious

  D. There are usually EEG changes

  E. They may respond to riboflavin

Exam 4: Answers

QUESTION 1

A. FALSE B. FALSE C. TRUE D. FALSE E. FALSE

A small VSD is often asymptomatic and most will close spontaneously during the first few years of life. The risk of endocarditis is not an indication for closure, though prophylaxis will be needed for certain procedures. The small VSDs have shorter louder systolic murmurs. A mid-diastolic apical murmur is heard with large defects. The ECG is normal and may show LVH if the murmur is large. If pulmonary hypertension develops, then RVH is seen on the ECG.

Surgical repair is indicated if there are severe symptoms with failure to thrive, if pulmonary hypertension develops, if aortic regurgitation develops, or if there is persistent significant shunting over 10 years of age.

QUESTION 2

A. TRUE B. FALSE C. FALSE D. FALSE E. FALSE

A supraventricular tachycardia (SVT) can be hard to distinguish from a ventricular tachycardia (VT).

Fusion and capture beats are seen in ventricular tachycardia.

AV association is present in SVT (dissociation in VT).

The heart rate may not be regular in SVT.

SVT responds to adenosine.

If there is uncertainty about the nature of the arrhythmia (SVT or VT?) then it should always be treated as VT.

QUESTION 3

A. TRUE B. FALSE C. FALSE D. TRUE E. TRUE

Peripheral pulmonary stenosis is seen in William's syndrome, congenital rubella syndrome and Alagille syndrome.

QUESTION 4

A. FALSE B. TRUE C. TRUE D. TRUE E. TRUE

A right sided aortic arch is seen in Fallot's tetralogy, truncus arteriosus, pulmonary atresia and commonly with a congenital vascular ring. It may also be present with no cardiac abnormality

QUESTION 5

A. FALSE B. TRUE C. TRUE D. TRUE E. FALSE

Pneumocystis carinii pneumonia in infants usually presents with an insidious onset of dyspnoea, tachypnoea, cough and fever at around 3 months in the immunocompromised infant. Septrin therapy can cause a neutropaenia, and also a rash. Bronchoalveolar lavage is necessary for diagnosis if sputum cannot be obtained otherwise. Hypoxia is a cardinal feature, and is often severe despite normal chest auscultation. The chest X-ray is normal in about 25% at presentation. Otherwise it shows perihilar shadowing 'butterfly rash', or a ground glass appearance with air bronchograms. Post-infection prophylaxis with septrin or pentamidine is recommended in the immunocompromised.

QUESTION 6

A. FALSE B. FALSE C. TRUE D. FALSE E. TRUE

Cystic adenomatoid malformation (CAM) of the lung is the second most common congenital lung malformation (congenital lobar emphysema being the most common). It usually causes a midline shift and compression of the opposite lung. It presents most commonly with neonatal respiratory distress, though may present with recurrent chest infections. Management is surgical with resection. There is no known association with Turner's syndrome.

QUESTION 7

A. TRUE B. TRUE C. FALSE D. TRUE E. FALSE

Nasal polyps in adults are more likely to signify aspirin sensitive asthma.

Staphylococcus aureus is the most common pathogen in infancy. After the age of 2 years the incidence of pseudomonas slowly rises.

Allergic bronchopulmonary aspergillosis is an allergic response to aspergillus, and therefore the treatment is steroids. The diagnosis is made by a combination of cough and wheeze, patchy shadowing on chest X-ray and a high specific IgE to Aspergillus.

QUESTION 8

A. FALSE B. TRUE C. FALSE D. TRUE E. FALSE

Anti-endomysial antibody is an IgA and as 1–4% of the general population have low IgA there may be a FALSE negative result in these individuals. A maximum pick up rate of giardia in the stools of 20% can be expected, and hence a trial of metronidazole for 5-7 days may be a better diagnostic tool. Primary lactase deficiency is rare, whereas post-gastroenteritis secondary lactase deficiency is not uncommon. Late onset congenital lactase deficiency occurs around the age of 10–14 especially in those of Mediterranean origin.

QUESTION 9

A. FALSE B. FALSE C. TRUE D. FALSE E. FALSE

Any nocturnal wakening with pain must be investigated for an organic cause. UTIs can occur without symptoms and an MSU is necessary in the majority of children with abdominal pain even if a psychogenic origin is suspected. Abdominal migraine occurs and usually has a preceding family history of classical migraine. There is no correlation, positive or negative between *H. pylori* serology and RAP of non-organic or organic origin.

Ref: Thomson M. Dyspepsia in childhood. In: *Baillière's Clinical Gastroenterology*. 1998.

QUESTION 10

A. FALSE B. TRUE C. TRUE D. FALSE E. FALSE

Toxic megacolon is a feature of ulcerative colitis. Terminal ileal involvement may cause a low vitamin B_{12}. Non-caseating granulomas occur. Until testicular volume is 20 ml there is still potential for increase in height. The warning area where urgent attention is necessary to treat the affected bowel to allow the pubertal growth spurt to occur is reached when testicular volume reaches 10 ml.

Ref: Leichtner A, Jackson W, Grand R. Chapter 27. In: *Pediatric Gastrointestinal Disease*. Ed Walker A. St Louis. 1996.

QUESTION 11

A. TRUE B. TRUE C. FALSE D. FALSE E. FALSE

Selenium stores are sufficient to account for requirements for 6 months when on a selenium-free diet (modern TPN will have selenium added to it), and deficiency can cause cardiomyopathy not pericarditis. Eggs, liver, and green vegetables are good sources of vitamin A.

QUESTION 12

A. TRUE B. TRUE C. TRUE D. TRUE E. FALSE

Atrial naturetic peptide also increases sodium and water excretion. It has no effect on vasoconstriction.

QUESTION 13

A. FALSE B. TRUE C. TRUE D. FALSE E. FALSE

In Type I mesangiocapillary GN a low C_3 and normal C_4 are classically observed with subendothelial immune complex deposition and splitting of the basement membrane. Type II results in mesangial cell proliferation and intramembranous immune complex deposition. Post-streptococcal GN (e.g. diffuse GN) may have low C_3 and normal C_4. Focal segmental, and rapidly progressive GN do not classically have complement decrease. Similarly membranous and minimal change do not have a low complement as a common feature.

QUESTION 14

A. FALSE B. TRUE C. TRUE D. FALSE E. FALSE

Proximal RTA is due to proximal tubule bicarbonate reabsorption, whereas distal RTA is due to distal tubule failure to excrete hydrogen ions. Rickets and aminoaciduria occur when associated with Fanconi's syndrome (Type II proximal RTA). Hyperchloraemia, hypokalaemia, low serum bicarbonate, and a metabolic acidosis with urine which can be acidified below pH 5.5, unlike distal RTA where the urine cannot be acidified below pH 5.8. Secondary causes of distal RTA include interstitial nephritis, obstructive nephropathy, and pyelonephritis.

QUESTION 15

A. FALSE B. TRUE C. TRUE D. TRUE E. FALSE

In some cases of UC, pANCA positivity may point towards multiple organ vaculitis and angiogram will reveal microaneurysms in the distribution of inferior mesenteric artery, renal bed, other visceral arterial supplies and even coronary arteries. Hamartomas or polycystic kidneys are associated with tuberous sclerosis. Hemihypertrophy may be associated with renal hyperplasia or Wilm's tumours.

QUESTION 16

A. TRUE   B. TRUE   C. FALSE   D. FALSE   E. FALSE

Liver biopsy usually distinguishes between neonatal hepatitis and biliary atresia but the two can still present with similar histological hepatic features – biliary duct hyperplasia is usually seen in biliary atresia and giant cells are typical of neonatal hepatitis. Phenobarbitone pre-administration prior to a liver isotope scan increases the likelihood of hepatobiliary excretion in neonatal hepatitis but not biliary atresia – it has no effect on uptake in either condition. If facial dysmorphism is seen with so-called "pinched facies" of hypertelorism, deep-set eyes, small mandible and a long nose then arterio-hepatic dysplasia, or Alagille's syndrome, should be suspected in the presence of jaundice. Biliary atresia is not characterised by jaundice in the first day of life as this is much more likely to be due to a haemolytic cause.

Ref: Davenport M and Howard E. Chapter 15. In: *Diseases of the liver and biliary system in childhood*. Ed Kelly D. Blackwell Science. Oxford 1999.

QUESTION 17

A. TRUE   B. FALSE   C. FALSE   D. TRUE   E. FALSE

After a 6 month course of 3-5 MIU/kg 3 times a week up to 40% of children will seroconvert to HBsAb and, where needed, HBeAb positive status, and may take up to 2 years after the end of the course to do so. HBsAg indicates carrier state, HBeAg indicates high infectivity, and HBsAb/HBeAb indicate seroconversion. In most studies no more than 1% of children go on to develop fulminant liver failure, the vast majority recovering without sequelae. 10% develop a chronic carrier state, of whom 10-30% remain asymptomatic and 70-90% develop cirrhosis - both situations can lead to hepatocellular carcinoma. HDV or delta virus exists solely in the HBsAg and is an incomplete RNA particle.

Ref: Davison S. Chapter 6. In: *Diseases of the liver and biliary system in childhood*. Ed Kelly D. Black-wellScience. Oxford 1999.

QUESTION 18

A. FALSE   B. FALSE   C. TRUE   D. FALSE   E. TRUE

Most hepatoblastomas occur under 18 months of age and HCC is commoner in older childhood. Short arm of chromosome 11 is implicated in the genetic aetiology of hepatoblastoma, and is associated with other embryonal tumours such as Wilms. Conversely, HCC seems to be associated with environmental factors. An abdominal mass will be present in 50-60% of HCCs and 70% of hepato-blastomas, but pain only occurs in 10-20%. Weight loss and anorexia are similarly uncommon (20%), and jaundice only appears in 7-10% of cases. MRI is the investigation of choice with further imaging of the vascularity by hepatic angiography if required. Calcification is not a feature.

Ref: Morland B and Buckels J. Chapter 16. In: *Diseases of the liver and biliary system in childhood*. Black-well Science. Oxford 1999.

QUESTION 19

A. FALSE   B. TRUE   C. FALSE   D. FALSE   E. FALSE

Although hypoglycaemia may occur in fulminant liver failure the commonest presentations are with symptoms such as nausea, anorexia and vomiting. Then, after 24-48 hours, right upper quadrant pain, followed by signs of overt hepatic injury at day 2-4. Normally it is conjugated to sulphate and glucuronide, but if this pathway is overwhelmed then the cytochrome P450 inducible system takes over and rapidly depletes the glutathione responsible for conjugating the toxic metabolites of this pathway from paracetamol. Hence enzyme induction will hasten toxicity. Paracetamol hepatotoxicity is a dose-dependent condition not reliant on hypersensitivity.

Ref: Davison S. Chapter 6. In: *Diseases of the liver and biliary system in childhood.* Ed Kelly D. Blackwell Science. Oxford 1999.

QUESTION 20

A. TRUE   B. TRUE   C. TRUE   D. TRUE   E. TRUE

In sideroblastic anaemia, hypochromic cells are seen in the peripheral blood, and ring sideroblasts are seen in the marrow with increased marrow iron (visible on Perls' reaction).

An inherited disease exists, which is X-linked recessive. Acquired disease may be primary (myelodysplsia FAB type 2) or secondary. Secondary disease is seen in malignant disease of the marrow, certain drugs (e.g. isoniazid), lead poisoning (basophilic stippling occurs), and haemolytic anaemia.

The blood film shows microcytic, hypochromic cells, and is often dimorphic. The bone marrow shows erythroblasts with a ring of iron granules in them, and increased iron deposition.

Management involves removing any treatable cause. Pyridoxine therapy may help, particularly in inherited disease. Folate therapy is given if deficiency is present. Repeated blood transfusions may be necessary.

QUESTION 21

A. TRUE   B. FALSE   C. TRUE   D. TRUE   E. FALSE

Diamond-Blackfan syndrome is an autosomal recessive condition. It is a red cell aplasia and presents as a severe anaemia by 2-6 months of age. A neutropaenia and a thrombocytosis may be present initially. The blood film shows a macrocytic anaemia with a young red cell population and reduced red cells. There are reduced red cell precursors in the bone marrow. Other abnormalities seen include triphalangeal thumbs, and dysmorphic facies.

QUESTION 22

A. TRUE   B. TRUE   C. FALSE   D. FALSE   E. TRUE

Idiopathic thrombocytopaenic purpura (ITP) is common in children. It usually occurs 1-4 weeks after a viral infection such as EBV, VZV and measles.

Clinical features are of bleeding with petechiae, bruises and mucosal bleeding. Intracranial haemorrhage occurs but is rare. Anti-platelet antibodies (both IgG and IgM) are seen. Most cases will resolve spontaneously in children, with only 5-10% becoming chronic.

Platelet transfusions are only given in emergency as they are quickly destroyed.

QUESTION 23

A. TRUE   B. FALSE   C. FALSE   D. TRUE   E. TRUE

The many causes of splenomegaly (useful to remember particularly for the clinical exam) may be classified into subgroups:

- Infectious causes e.g. EBV, subacute bacterial endocarditis, and brucellosis
- Extramedullary haemopoiesis e.g. haemolytic anaemias, haemoglobinopathies, osteopetrosis
- Congestion e.g. portal hypertension
- Neoplastic conditions e.g. leukaemia
- Storage diseases e.g. Neimann-Pick disease, Gaucher's disease, LCH, mucopolysaccharidoses
- Other systemic diseases e.g. amyloidosis, SLE
- Massive splenomegaly is classically seen in malaria, kalar-Azar, CML and myelofibrosis

QUESTION 24

A. FALSE   B. TRUE   C. FALSE   D. FALSE   E. TRUE

Wilms' tumour is associated with neurofibromatosis, hemihypertrophy, aniridia, genitourinary anomalies and Beckwith-Weidemann syndrome.

QUESTION 25

A. FALSE   B. FALSE   C. TRUE   D. FALSE   E. TRUE

The factors associated with a **good** prognosis in ALL are:

- Female sex
- Low initial WCC
- Age 2-10 years
- Less than 4 weeks to initial remission
- Translocation 12:21
- Hyperdiploidy
- c-ALL

The other features in the question are associated with a **poor** prognosis.

QUESTION 26

A. FALSE   B. TRUE   C. TRUE   D. FALSE   E. TRUE

IgG is present at adult levels at birth due to placental transfer of the immunoglobulin. The levels fall off during the first few months and reach lowest levels at 3-6 months before climbing slowly to reach adult levels by 5-6 years. This may result in transient hypogammaglobulinaemia of infancy. IgA is absent at birth and levels slowly rise to reach adult levels by puberty. IgM is also absent at birth with adult levels being reached by about 1 year of age. If there are increased levels of IgM at birth, this indicates intra-uterine infection.

QUESTION 27

A. TRUE   B. FALSE   C. TRUE   D. TRUE   E. TRUE

Ataxia telangiectasia involves both impaired cell mediated immunity and impaired antibody production. In particular, IgA is very low. IgE and IgG_2 and IgG_4 are also low. There is a defect in DNA repair, and an extreme sensitivity to ionising radiation. The genetic defect involves mutations in the ATM gene on chromosome 11. Both serum AFP and CEA are elevated.

QUESTION 28

A. FALSE   B. TRUE   C. FALSE   D. TRUE   E. TRUE

Patients with a history of anaphylaxis to eggs should not receive the egg-based vaccines: MMR, influenza and yellow fever.

N.B. MMR vaccination should only take place where resuscitation facilities are available (e.g. in a hospital paediatric unit).

QUESTION 29

A. FALSE   B. FALSE   C. FALSE   D. TRUE   E. TRUE

Measles is infectious in the pre-eruptive stage, not the eruptive stage. Forchheimer spots are palatal petechiae which are classically seen in Rubella.

The incubation period is short (7-14 days). Koplik spots are small grey lesions on the gums next to the 2nd molar and they are pathognomonic.

EEG abnormalities are seen in the acute disease in around 50% of cases.

QUESTION 30

A. FALSE   B. FALSE   C. TRUE   D. FALSE   E. TRUE

Lyme disease is caused by the spirochaete, *Borellia burgdorfei*, and is transmitted by Ixodid ticks on deer and sheep. The diagnosis is by measuring the IgM antibodies. The first feature is Erythema chronicum migrans (a painless red rash, spreading outwards). Most cases will develop a chronic arthritis within months to years without treatment.

QUESTION 31

A. FALSE   B. FALSE   C. FALSE   D. TRUE   E. TRUE

Rabies enters via the bite, replicates in the muscle locally and spreads via the peripheral nerves to the brain where it replicates further.

The vaccine is a killed organism vaccine.

Rabies has an incubation period of 1-3 months on average, though it may be much longer.

Aerophobia is pathognomonic, but hydrophobia is seen in around half of cases.

Dumb rabies is a form involving a symmetrical ascending paralysis and is spread by bats.

QUESTION 32

A. TRUE   B. FALSE   C. TRUE   D. FALSE   E. FALSE

Acute haemorrhagic conjunctivitis may be caused by enteroviral infection, with enterovirus 70 identified in epidemics. Adenovirus classically causes epidemic conjunctivitis.

Ludwig's angina is a diffuse infection of the submandibular and sublingual spaces, and is usually bacterial.

Coxsackie A and B are the most common causes of Herpangina.

The enteroviruses include Poliovirus, Coxsackie viruses A and B, echoviruses and enteroviruses.

Coxsackie A16 is the major cause of hand foot and mouth disease.

QUESTION   33

A. TRUE   B. TRUE   C. FALSE   D. FALSE   E. TRUE

Urea cycle defects are a group of disorders involving defects of metabolism of ammonia in the urea cycle. They include carbamylphosphate synthetase deficiency (CPS), ornithine transcarbamylase deficiency (OTC), arginosuccinate synthatase (AS) deficiency, arginosuccinate lyase (AL) deficiency, arginase deficiency and N-acetylglutamate synthetase deficiency.

Initial investigations include a significantly raised serum ammonia level (usually > 200 μmol/l). Plasma amino acid profile and urine orotic acid analysis usually make the initial diagnosis, which is confirmed by enzyme analysis.

Long-term management is with dietary protein restriction, avoidance of catabolic states and individual supplements.

QUESTION   34

A. TRUE   B. FALSE   C. TRUE   D. FALSE   E. TRUE

Chondrodysplasia punctata is a stippled appearance of the epiphyses of bones which is apparent on X-ray. It is seen in a number of conditions including:

- Zellweger syndrome (a peroxisomal disorder)
- Rhizomelic chondrodysplasia punctata
- Warfarin toxicity
- Conradi–Hunermann syndrome

QUESTION   35

A. TRUE   B. FALSE   C. TRUE   D. FALSE   E. TRUE

First line investigations in a metabolic screen can include:

- Serum: Urea and electrolytes, glucose, ketones, ammonia, liver function tests, clotting screen, lactate and amino acids
- Blood gas
- Urine: Organic acids and ketones
- CSF: Lactate and glycine

Enzyme analysis is required for definitive diagnosis.

QUESTION   36

A. TRUE   B. FALSE   C. FALSE   D. FALSE   E. TRUE

Noonan syndrome and XY/XO mosaicism (Turner syndrome mosaicism) both cause short stature. XYY does not result in short stature, and neither does testicular feminisation syndrome (now less confusingly known as androgen insensitivity syndrome). Chronic illness results in proportionate short stature. Disproportionate short stature is seen in bone dyscrasias, for example, achondroplasia.

QUESTION   37

A. TRUE   B. FALSE   C. FALSE   D. TRUE   E. TRUE

Polycystic ovary syndrome is a condition involving multiple small ovarian cysts and hormonal imbalance. The clinical features include secondary amenorrhoea or menstrual irregularity, hirsutism, obesity, acne and infertility. Osteoporosis is not a feature. There is mild hyperprolactinaemia, and a raised LH level, with a raised LH:FSH level. Testosterone levels are moderately raised and may be normal.

The oral contraceptive pill may help, and the anti-androgen cyproterone may be used.

QUESTION   38

A. FALSE   B. FALSE   C. TRUE   D. FALSE   E. TRUE

Type 1 diabetes mellitus most commonly presents in older children, though can occur at any age. It most commonly presents in the Spring and Autumn. About 80% of children have islet cell antibodies on first presentation. The disease is associated wth HLA B8, DR3 and DR4.

Siblings have a 1 in 20 chance of developing the disease. The risk for a child developing the disease is increased if a parent has it, and the risk is greater if the father has it.

QUESTION   39

A. TRUE   B. TRUE   C. FALSE   D. TRUE   E. TRUE

Infants of diabetic mothers have a 3 times increased risk of congenital malformations. In particular they may have macrosomia, hypoplastic left colon, sacral agenesis and congenital heart disease. The neonate is at increased risk of respiratory distress syndrome, polycythaemia and hypoglycaemia.

QUESTION   40

A. TRUE   B. FALSE   C. TRUE   D. FALSE   E. TRUE

Aniridia may be inherited as autosomal dominant, with chromosome 2p or chromosome 11p deletions. It may be also be inherited as autosomal recessive, and about a third of cases are sporadic. Cataract is often associated and visual acuity is markedly reduced. There may be nystagmus and macular hypoplasia. There is a strong association with Wilms tumour, both in the inherited chromosome 11p deletion and in the sporadic forms, and therefore screening with renal ultrasound scans is necessary.

QUESTION   41

A. TRUE   B. FALSE   C. FALSE   D. FALSE   E. FALSE

Absence seizures if typical last less than 30 seconds, are not preceded by an aura and do not have a post-ictal state. Complex absence seizures may have a motor component such as myotonic movements.

A 3 per second spike and wave pattern is seen on the EEG.

QUESTION   42

A. TRUE   B. TRUE   C. FALSE   D. TRUE   E. FALSE

Acute cerebellar ataxia may be caused by varicella infection as a post-infectious event and phenytoin therapy where it is a sign of toxicity. A cerebellar tumour may result in acute ataxia if there is a bleed into it, though usually it is a cause of chronic ataxia. Joubert disease and Abetalipoproteinaemia are causes of chronic ataxia, the latter secondary to vitamin E deficiency.

QUESTION 43

A. FALSE   B. FALSE   C. TRUE   D. FALSE   E. TRUE

In myaesthenia gravis, edrophonium is used to diagnose the condition, and results in a short-lived relief from the symptoms. The external ocular muscles are affected and there is diploplia and a partial ptosis. It is associated with HLA-B8, DR3. There are IgG antibodies to acetylcholine receptors. Infants may develop a transient form of the condition as the antibodies cross the placenta.

QUESTION 44

A. FALSE   B. TRUE   C. FALSE   D. TRUE   E. TRUE

Legg-Clave-Perthes disease is one of the osteochondritides. It involves aseptic necrosis of the femoral head. It is 5 times more common in males. It is bilateral in around a fifth of cases. Children under 6 years are generally managed conservatively, while those over 6 are managed with exercises and bed rest, abduction casts and osteotomy if necessary.

QUESTION 45

A. FALSE   B. FALSE   C. TRUE   D. FALSE   E. FALSE

Activated charcoal is not of proven benefit, but stomach washout can be helpful. Apparent early clinical recovery may lead to a false sense of security, as later degeneration can occur. Pyloric stenosis can occur 2-4 weeks later as a result of scarring from local irritation. Hepatic necrosis can occur but if it does it takes 2-4 days for the cytochrome enzymes to cease to function, and for cell death to ensue. Oral desferrioxamine should not be given as it may theoretically increase iron absorption and is expensive.

QUESTION 46

A. FALSE   B. TRUE   C. FALSE   D. TRUE   E. FALSE

Intravenous diazepam is effective for only 20-30 minutes (i.e. enough time for phenytoin to be given). A recent study in the USA found that phenytoin appears to reduce cognitive function more than carbamazepine or sodium valproate. There is an estimated 10% risk of the foetal hydantoin syndrome (craniofacial and limb abnormalities) in infants of women on chronic phenytoin therapy. However, a severe agranulocytosis and aplastic anaemia is seen in 1 in 500 000. Absence seizures are managed with ethosuximide and sodium valproate.

QUESTION 47

A. TRUE   B. TRUE   C. TRUE   D. FALSE   E. TRUE

Dopamine has a short half-life and therefore an infusion is necessary. A plateau is reached by 5 half-lives (i.e. about 10 minutes). It increases renal blood flow via dopamine receptors on the renal arteries. Alkaline, not acidic, solutions such as bicarbonate will inactivate dopamine.

QUESTION 48

A. FALSE   B. TRUE   C. FALSE   D. TRUE   E. FALSE

Bone marrow suppression starts at around 7 days and peaks at 10-14 days, returning to normal within 21-28 days. A polyneuropathy is typically seen, although SIADH, autonomic dysfunction and cortical blindness are all reported. Vincristine is extremely toxic to tissues and extravasation requires urgent action. Pain, swelling and poor blood return should be looked for. Vincristine binds to the mitotic spindle during the M-phase causing its termination. Vincristine is metabolised via the liver and therefore the dose should be reduced in biliary tract disease.

QUESTION 49

A. FALSE B. FALSE C. FALSE D. FALSE E. TRUE

Waardenberg syndrome involves partial albinism, not vitiligo. The albinism usually involves a white forelock and pale blue or heterochromic irises. The hair may become prematurely grey or white. Deafness is present in 25% of Type I cases, and 50% of Type II cases.

The disorder has been classified into Type I (including lateral displacement of the inner canthi) caused by mutations in the PAX3 gene on chromosome 2q35. And Type II (no inner canthi displacement) caused by mutations in the human microphthalmia gene at chromosome 3p12.3-14.1. Both types are of autosomal dominant inheritance.

Hirschsprung's disease may be associated, along with oesophageal and anal atresia.

QUESTION 50

A. TRUE B. TRUE C. TRUE D. FALSE E. FALSE

Systemic-onset JCA is of equal sex incidence and may occur at any age of childhood. It is a clinical diagnosis, and the differential diagnoses include lymphoma, other malignancies, vasculitis, infection and other connective tissue diseases.

Clinical features are intermittent fevers, a variable rash which is classically salmon-pink, however, myalgia, arthralgia, hepatosplenomegaly and lymphadenopathy. Pericardial effusions may occur. A polyarthritis occurs within a few months of disease onset in around half of cases. Late features do include amyloidosis, as well as short stature and micrognathia.

ANA and RhF are negative.

QUESTION 51

A. FALSE B. FALSE C. TRUE D. TRUE E. TRUE

Juvenile onset dermatomyositis is a multisystem disease with inflammation of striated muscle and cutaneous lesions. The HLA associations include B8, DR3 and DQA1*0501. If untreated, the mortality is high (up to 40%) but if treated, it is around 2-5%, though many (30-40%) will remain disabled. Clinical features include muscle pain with proximal muscle weakness and dysphagia, palatal regurgitation and respiratory muscle weakness. Cutaneous features include the heliotrope rash over the eyelids which is pathognomonic. Nail fold capillaries are also seen (look hard for these), and Grotton papules (red lumps over the DIP, PIP and knee joints). A butterfly rash over the face may be seen and subcutaneous calcium deposits may occur and these may extrude. Other features include joint involvement (arthralgia, arthritis and contractures), gastrointestinal (ulcerations and bleeding), myocarditis, nephritis, CNS disease, interstitial lung disease, pulmonary haemorrhage, hepatosplenomegaly and retinitis.

QUESTION 52

A. TRUE B. FALSE C. FALSE D. TRUE E. FALSE

Blue sclerae are seen in a number of diseases, involving defects in collagen. These include Ehlers-Danlos syndrome, Marfan's syndrome, Pseudoxanthoma elasticum and osteogenesis imperfecta types I, II and III (type III variable).

In phenylketonuria, blue irises are seen if the disease is untreated.

QUESTION 53

A. FALSE B. FALSE C. TRUE D. TRUE E. TRUE

The polymerase chain reaction (PCR) is a technique to rapidly make millions of copies of DNA which can then be used for analysis. It makes it possible to analyse DNA from very small samples of blood (i.e. a blood stain which may be several years old). PCR can be employed in antenatal chorionic villous sampling to enable rapid diagnosis (diagnosis in one day rather than one week). PCR cannot amplify very long sequences, and thus cannot be used to detect very large deletions.

The technique of PCR involves heating genomic DNA to denature it and produce single strands. Then the DNA is exposed to primer sequences which anneal to the complementary base pairs as the DNA is cooled to an annealing temperature. These primers flank the region of interest. The reaction is then heated to an intermediate temperature, and the primer sequence is extended as base pairs are added by DNA polymerase. This double stranded DNA is heated again to denature it. The heating-cooling cycle is repeated, and the newly formed DNA acts as a template for further DNA formation. Thus the number of copies doubles in each cycle by a chain reaction, and millions of copies of the original DNA are formed after several repeat cycles.

QUESTION 54

A. TRUE B. FALSE C. TRUE D. TRUE E. FALSE

Trinucleotide repeat expansion is seen in some inherited conditions, and successive generations may become more severely affected as the expansion occurs. The diseases associated with trinucleotide repeat expansions include:

Huntington's disease, spinocerebellar ataxia types 1, 2, 3 and 6 (CAG repeat sequence, expansion occurs more often through the father) and myotonic dystrophy (CTG) and Fragile X syndrome (CGG) (expansion through the mother), and Friedreich's ataxia (GAA repeat sequence, expansion through either parent).

Miller-Deiker is is a microdeletion syndrome of chromosomal deletion 17p13.3.

MERRF is a mitochodrial DNA mutation disease.

QUESTION 55

A. FALSE B. TRUE C. TRUE D. FALSE E. TRUE

Trisomy 21 (Down's syndrome) has an overall incidence of 1:650. The risk increases with maternal age, with an incidence of 1:100 to those of age 40 years. The genetic causes are non-disjunction (95%), Robertsonian translocation (4%) and mosaicism (1%).

Variable recurrence risk is seen, depending on the cause, and for this reason it is essential that chromosome studies are done.

For non-disjunction, the risk of recurrence is 1:200 if mother < 35 years, and twice the age specific rate if mother > 35 years.

In Robertsonian translocation the recurrence risk is 10-15% if the mother is the carrier, and 2.5% if the father is the carrier. The risk is 100% if a parent carries the translocation 21:21. The risk is < 1% if neither parent carries a translocation.

Hypotonia is a consistent feature in infancy, occuring in approximately 80% of babies, and improving with age. Cardiac anomalies occur in 40% of infants. The commonest type is AVSD, then VSD, then PDA and then ASD.

QUESTION 56

A. FALSE B. FALSE C. FALSE D. TRUE E. TRUE

- The paired t-test is used to compare two dependant samples
- The Mann-Whitney test is used on non-parametric data
- The unpaired t-test is used on parametric data
- Wilcoxon is the equivalent of the paired t-test used on non-parametric data
- The Chi-squared test may be used on frequencies obtained from parametric or non-parametric data

QUESTION 57

A. FALSE B. TRUE C. FALSE D. FALSE E. TRUE

Erb's palsy results from damage to the upper nerve roots (C5 and C6) of the brachial plexus. The arm is held in abduction, with the elbow extended, the forearm pronated and the wrist flexed (the 'waiters tip' position). A wrist drop occurs in Klumpke's palsy. Most, but not all, will recover fully after several months. Physiotherapy is necessary, and prevents contractures developing.

QUESTION 58

A. TRUE B. TRUE C. TRUE D. TRUE E. TRUE

Infants of maternal drug abusers show many signs of drug withdrawal for which they need to be monitored and managed. Increased lacrimation and rhinorrhea are features of drug withdrawal. These infants have an increased basal metabolic rate. They are managed with conservative measures which include decreased sensory stimuli, frequent feeds and swaddling. Drug treatment may be with opiates and sedatives as necessary. These infants are at increased risk of SIDS.

QUESTION 59

A. FALSE B. TRUE C. FALSE D. TRUE E. TRUE

Unconjugated neonatal hyperbilirubinaemia may be caused by Gilbert's syndrome, Hirschsprung's disease and galactosaemia. Biliary atresia and Alagille syndrome cause conjugated hyperbilirubinaemia.

QUESTION 60

A. FALSE B. TRUE C. FALSE D. FALSE E. FALSE

Neonatal seizures are often difficult to recognise, and may present simply as apnoea. One way of differentiating them from jitteriness is that they do not stop if the limb is held. Myoclonic seizures are concerning as they often indicate a severe underlying abnormality.

Most neonatal seizures are not obviously associated with EEG changes. A few seizures will be due to pyridoxine deficiency and respond to its replacement.

Exam 5: Questions

QUESTION 1

An ostium primum ASD

- **A.** Results in right axis deviation (RAD) on the ECG
- **B.** Is seen in Holt–Oram syndrome
- **C.** Is the most common form of ASD
- **D.** May be left to close spontaneously
- **E.** Reverse splitting of the 2nd heart sound occurs

QUESTION 2

In Wolf–Parkinson–White (WPW) syndrome

- **A.** There is a risk of ventricular tachycardia
- **B.** Presentation may be with hydrops foetalis
- **C.** Type a is seen in association with Ebstein's anomaly
- **D.** Flecanide reduces the recurrence risk of tachycardias
- **E.** The ECG shows a narrow QRS complex

QUESTION 3

In Tetralogy of Fallot

- **A.** Cyanosis is reduced by taking a hot bath
- **B.** Cyanosis is often present in the first few days of life
- **C.** There is a right sided aortic arch in about 50% of cases
- **D.** The murmur becomes softer during a cyanotic spell as flow through the pulmonary valve is increased
- **E.** There is an association with DiGeorge syndrome

QUESTION 4

Regarding infective endocarditis

- **A.** It is commonly seen with atrial septal defects
- **B.** It can be associated with aneurysms of the cerebral arteries
- **C.** Osler's nodes are commonly seen
- **D.** Splinter haemorrhages are present in about 25% of cases
- **E.** It is caused by staphylococcus aureus in about half of the cases of acute endocarditis

QUESTION 5

Lymphocytic interstitial pneumonitis (LIP)

A. Is uncommon in vertically acquired HIV infection
B. Is due to a protozoal infection
C. Is seen on chest X-ray as a perihilar infiltration in a 'butterfly distribution'
D. May be associated with hepatosplenomegaly
E. Steroid therapy is always necessary

QUESTION 6

In cystic fibrosis

A. The underlying defect lies in sodium channel function
B. The immune reactive trypsin (IRT) may be checked on the Guthrie card
C. In most cases the genetic defect is a loss of valine at position 508 on chromosome 7
D. A sweat test with a sodium content above 40 mmol/l is diagnostic
E. A false positive sweat test may be seen in ectodermal dysplasia

QUESTION 7

Regarding severe respiratory compromise

A. Subcostal and intercostal recession are more significant signs of respiratory compromise in infants than in school age children
B. Respiratory failure is second only to cardiac failure as the commonest cause of cardiac arrest in children
C. The loudness of the inspiratory wheeze corresponds directly with the severity of the bronchospasm
D. In respiratory failure treatment should only be given after thorough examination
E. Oxygen given via nasal cannulae results in a constant inspired oxygen concentration

QUESTION 8

Associations of coeliac disease include

A. Epilepsy with posterior cerebellar calcification
B. IgA nephropathy
C. Oesophageal carcinoma
D. Addison's disease
E. Sjögren's syndrome

QUESTION 9

Hirschsprung's disease

A. Is inherited in an autosomal recessive fashion
B. Is due to unopposed parasympathetic activity in the affected segment of the bowel
C. Has an equal incidence in girls and boys
D. Is seen more frequently in children with Down's syndrome than in the general population
E. Presents in more than 80% in the neonatal period

QUESTION 10

The following more commonly occur in Crohn's disease than ulcerative colitis

- **A.** Erythema nodosum
- **B.** Pyoderma gangrenosum
- **C.** Ankylosing spondyloarthropathy with HLA B27
- **D.** Uveitis
- **E.** Cholangiocarcinoma

QUESTION 11

Anorexia nervosa

- **A.** Is more common than bulimia
- **B.** Can have a low T_4 in the presence of a normal T_3
- **C.** Can demonstrate a raised growth hormone
- **D.** May have a hypochloraemic hypokalaemic alkalosis
- **E.** Is associated with diarrhoea more commonly than constipation

QUESTION 12

The following are causes of haematuria in childhood

- **A.** Alport's syndrome
- **B.** *E. coli* 0157
- **C.** Factor V Leiden deficiency
- **D.** α thalassaemia
- **E.** Rapid increase in intracranial pressure

QUESTION 13

Henoch-Schönlein purpura

- **A.** Has a preponderance for late Winter and early Summer
- **B.** Exhibits a male:female ratio of 2:1
- **C.** Is associated with a raised IgA in over 40%
- **D.** May cause death from pulmonary haemorrhage
- **E.** Is associated with a prolonged bleeding time

QUESTION 14

Fanconi's syndrome

- **A.** Is associated with cystinuria
- **B.** Is usually associated with a haemoglobin < 10g/dl
- **C.** Results in dehydration, polyuria and polydipsia
- **D.** Is acquired by glue-sniffing
- **E.** Can produce a urine with a pH of 5.0 and a metabolic acidosis

QUESTION 15

In a child with minimal change nephrotic syndrome

A. Penicillamine is a recognised cause
B. A history in the previous 6 weeks of a streptococcal illness is likely
C. The albumin:creatinine ratio is > 200 mg/mmol
D. Initial management is prednisolone 90 mg/m²/day
E. Abdominal pain requires parenteral penicillin and a watch and wait policy

QUESTION 16

In Alagille's syndrome the features which are recognised include

A. Tuberous xanthomas and raised serum cholesterol
B. Progression to cirrhosis and chronic liver failure requiring liver transplant
C. Tubulointerstitial nephropathy
D. Tetralogy of Fallot
E. Abnormalities of peroxisomal function

QUESTION 17

In paediatric liver disease portal hypertension

A. Occurs when portal pressure is elevated to 10-12 mmHg
B. Results in cephalic flow of collaterals inferior to the umbilicus
C. May cause signs of spinal compression
D. May result from Factor V Leiden deficiency
E. Should be treated prophylactically with propranolol under the age of 12 years

QUESTION 18

In acute liver failure

A. Aminotransferase levels are not predictive of outcome
B. Due to sodium valproate therapy the chance for a neurologically intact outcome is very poor
C. Hyperventilation usually accompanies stage II-III hepatic encephalopathy and may result in respiratory alkalosis
D. Fluid restriction to <75% of maintenance is the key strategy in prevention of intracerebral oedema
E. Coagulation support should only be used if active bleeding occurs or to cover invasive procedures

QUESTION 19

In chronic liver disease in childhood the following are correct

A. Spironolactone is useful in the treatment of ascites at any age
B. A low plasma cholesterol is an adverse prognostic feature
C. Sleep reversal occurs as a feature of hepatic encephalopathy
D. There is an increased overall incidence of Hirschsprung's disease
E. Spontaneous bacterial peritonitis is a potentially fatal complication of ascites

QUESTION   20

The following are features found in intravascular haemolysis

A. Red cell fragments
B. Haemoglobinaemia
C. Haemosiderinuria
D. Haemoglobinuria
E. Methaemoglobinaemia

QUESTION   21

Features of homozygous sickle cell disease include

A. Dactylitis
B. Presentation usually during the first few months of life
C. Increased incidence of Salmonella osteomyelitis
D. Proliferative retinopathy
E. Pigment gallstones

QUESTION   22

A prolonged bleeding time is seen in

A. von Willebrand's disease
B. Bernard-Soulier syndrome
C. Glanzmann's disease
D. Hermansky-Pudlak syndrome
E. Haemophilia B

QUESTION   23

The following are causes of neonatal thrombocytopaenia

A. Bernard-Soulier syndrome
B. Congenital rubella infection
C. Leukaemia
D. Renal vein thrombosis
E. Giant haemangioma

QUESTION   24

Osteosarcoma

A. Is a small round cell neoplasm
B. Has a predeliction for the flat bones
C. Is associated with retinoblastoma
D. Is less common than Ewing's sarcoma
E. X-ray findings include lytic lesions

QUESTION 25

In acute myeloid leukaemia (AML)

A. Gum hypertrophy is a clinical feature of the M4 and M5 subtypes
B. Fanconi syndrome is associated
C. Auer rods are always seen
D. DIC is a feature of the M3 (acute promyelocytic) subtype
E. Retinoic acid may be used as initial therapy in the M2 subtype

QUESTION 26

Bruton's X-linked agammaglobulinaemia

A. Involves a mutation in the btk gene
B. Is inherited as autosomal recessive
C. Is associated with unusual entroviral infections
D. A block is present in the maturation of pre-B cells
E. Usually presents with *pneumocystis carinii* pneumonia

QUESTION 27

In Job's syndrome

A. IgM counts are very high
B. It is due to mutations in the intracellular kinase Jak 3
C. Eczema is a feature
D. Small platelets are seen
E. Recurrent staphylococcal skin abscesses occur

QUESTION 28

The Haemophilus influenza b vaccine

A. Is composed of the polysaccharide coat and a protein
B. Provides protection against non-encapsulated organisms
C. Protects against epiglottitis
D. Is a live vaccine
E. Is effective in the neonate

QUESTION 29

Mumps

A. Is a DNA virus
B. Is a common cause of viral meningitis
C. Involves purely the submandibular gland in 20% of cases
D. Is a cause of pancreatitis
E. May cause myocarditis

QUESTION 30

Concerning malaria

A. *Plasmodium vivax* infects only the old red blood cells
B. Nephrotic syndrome can be seen in *Plasmodium malariae* infection
C. *Plasmodium falciparum* has a latent phase in the liver
D. Sporozoites rupture to release merozoites in the blood
E. Primaquine is needed for eradication in *Plasmodium malariae*

QUESTION 31

Regarding leprosy

A. The incubation period is 1-3 months
B. The lepromin test is negative in Lepromatous leprosy
C. The diagnosis is by culturing the organism in artificial media
D. The clinical disease is dependant on the immune status of the individual
E. Tuberculoid leprosy is seen in people with poor cell-mediated immunity

QUESTION 32

In bacterial meningitis

A. CSF glucose:plasma ratio is high
B. Approximately one fifth of infants will present with seizures
C. Subdural effusions are rare
D. Kernig sign is almost always positive
E. Rifampicin is given to contacts of *S. pneumoniae* meningitis

QUESTION 33

In galactosaemia

A. There is an incidence of 1 in 6 000
B. The enzyme deficiency is of glucose phosphorylase
C. There is an inability to metabolise galactose and lactose
D. Diagnosis is by red blood cell enzyme assay
E. Speech problems are almost inevitable even with therapy

QUESTION 34

The mitochondrial disorders

A. May present at any age and by any mode of inheritance
B. Include Pearson's syndrome
C. Features may include retinitis pigmentosa
D. Include myoclinic epilepsy and ragged-red fibres (MERRF)
E. Elevated free-floating blood lactate supports the diagnosis

QUESTION 35

X-linked adrenoleucodystrophy

A. Is a mitochondrial disorder
B. May present as Addison's disease
C. Involves accumulation of short chain fatty acids
D. Involves progressive neuronal white matter degeneration
E. Lorenzo's oil is curative

QUESTION 36

In congenital hypothyroidism

A. Ectopic thyroid tissue is the commonest finding
B. Dyshormonogenesis accounts for around 25%
C. The incidence is around 1 in 6000
D. May result from maternal hyperthyroidism
E. Significant intellectual impairment is inevitable

QUESTION 37

The following may result in diabetes insipidus

A. Craniopharyngioma
B. Carbamazepine
C. Demeclocycline
D. Neonatal listeriosis
E. The DIDMOAD syndrome

QUESTION 38

Craniopharyngioma

A. Is one of the most common infratentorial tumours in childhood
B. May present with tall stature
C. May present with polyuria
D. Arises from a remnant of the connection between Rathke's pouch and the oral cavity
E. Is associated with calcification on the skull X-ray in about 20%

QUESTION 39

In familial hypophosphataemic rickets

A. There is defective distal renal tubule reabsorption of phosphate
B. Levels of 1,25 dihydroxycholecalciferol are normal
C. Parathyroid hormone levels are raised
D. Plasma calcium levels are high
E. The inheritance is autosomal dominant

QUESTION 40

Children high on the autistic spectrum

- **A.** Demonstrate repetitive behaviour
- **B.** Have distinctive abnormal findings on the EEG
- **C.** Have delayed motor milestones
- **D.** Have a good emotional contact with the mother but not with any strangers
- **E.** Have normal speech development

QUESTION 41

Febrile convulsions

- **A.** Occur in 8-10% of children
- **B.** Are more common in males than females
- **C.** Typically occur between 6 months and 6 years
- **D.** Are not associated with increased risk of later development of epilepsy
- **E.** Are usually associated with a positive family history

QUESTION 42

Features of Late Infantile Batten Disease include

- **A.** Acute intermittent ataxia
- **B.** Developmental regression
- **C.** Diagnosis on rectal biopsy
- **D.** X-linked recessive inheritance
- **E.** Retinitis pigmentosa

QUESTION 43

In raised intracranial pressure

- **A.** Drowsiness is seen with a rapidly increasing pressure
- **B.** Convulsions are a common presentation
- **C.** The headache is worse on movement
- **D.** There may be a sixth nerve palsy
- **E.** Signs take longer to develop in young children than in adults

QUESTION 44

Slipped upper femoral epiphysis

- **A.** Is seen in children age 5-10 years most commonly
- **B.** Is associated with hypothyroidism
- **C.** May present with knee pain
- **D.** Is seen on hip X-ray with a narrowing of the growth plate
- **E.** Shows decreased external rotation of the hip on examination

QUESTION 45

The following concerning antimalarials are true

A. Chloroquine is always contraindicated in G6PD deficiency
B. Proguanil inhibits folate production
C. Mefloquine causes neuropsychiatric symptoms in up to 10% of patients
D. Pyrimethamine resisitance is low
E. Long term chloroquine is associated with cataract

QUESTION 46

Doxorubicin

A. Is an anthracycline
B. Is more effective against solid tumours than daunorubicin
C. Is cardiotoxic to all patients
D. Binds to DNA
E. Is safe in patients with a history of shingles

QUESTION 47

Liver enzyme inducers include

A. Carbamazepine
B. Rifampicin
C. Brussel sprouts
D. Phenytoin
E. Tobacco smoke

QUESTION 48

The following are true of salicylate poisoning

A. Hypokalaemia is a feature
B. Hypoventilation is an early feature
C. Vasodilation is a feature
D. Coma indicates severe poisoning
E. Respiratory alkalosis is seen in children

QUESTION 49

Mollusca contagiosa

A. Is caused by a pox virus
B. Is seen as a pearly papule with a central umbilicus
C. Spontaneous resolution is usual by 6 weeks
D. May be disseminated in a child with atopic eczema
E. May be treated with cryotherapy

QUESTION 50

Reiter's syndrome

A. Is associated with *Campylobacter* gastroenteritis
B. Responds well to antibiotics
C. Keratoderma blenorrhagica may be a feature
D. Usually resolves within a year of onset
E. Does not become chronic

QUESTION 51

Regarding Kawasaki disease

A. It is a polyarteritis
B. A fever of > 37.5°C should be present for 5 days to make the diagnosis
C. Untreated, nearly 2% of children will develop coronary artery aneurysms
D. Intravenous immunoglobulin should be given within 3 weeks of onset of disease
E. A marked thrombocytopaenia is seen in the second and third week of disease

QUESTION 52

Syndromes involving absent radii include

A. Stickler's dysplasia
B. Holt-Oram syndrome
C. Ellis-Van Creveld syndrome
D. Fanconi anaemia
E. VATER syndrome

QUESTION 53

Features of Noonan syndrome include

A. Peripheral pulmonary stenosis
B. Ventricular septal defect
C. Ptosis
D. Mental retardation
E. Autosomal dominant inheritance

QUESTION 54

In embryological development of the lung

A. The lung bud is an outgrowth of the midgut
B. The respiratory bronchioles develop from 22 weeks gestation
C. The lung bud derives from mesodermal tissue
D. Type I pneumocytes produce surfactant
E. Surfactant production can be detected by 23 weeks gestation

QUESTION   55

Multifactorial inheritance

A. Is seen in the inheritance of pyloric stenosis
B. Involves both genetic and environmental factors
C. Means that the inheritance risk for relatives cannot be estimated
D. Operates in the inheritance of neural tube defects
E. Risks for multifactorial inheritance increase if more family members are affected

QUESTION   56

The following are true

A. A single blind trial indicates that neither the patient nor the assessor know which group a patient has been assigned to
B. The Chi-squared test is carried out using percentages
C. Randomisation will help eliminate selection bias
D. The median is the value which occurs most often
E. The incidence of a disorder is the number of the population suffering from a disorder at one point in time

QUESTION   57

Human breast milk

A. Contains less carbohydrate than cow's milk
B. Contains less iron than cow's milk
C. Is associated with an increased risk of haemorrhagic disease of the newborn
D. Has a higher casein to whey ratio than cow's milk
E. Has more protein than cow's milk

QUESTION   58

The following conditions are associated with delayed closure of the anterior fontanelle

A. Achondroplasia
B. Apert syndrome
C. Hyperthryroidism
D. Progeria
E. Malnutrition

QUESTION   59

The following may result in neonatal hypocalcaemia

A. Infant of a diabetic mother
B. Birth asphyxia
C. Infant fed on high-phosphate cow's milk formula
D. Hypermagnasaemia
E. Neonatal hyperparathyroidism

QUESTION 60

In twin pregnancy

A. In twin-twin transfusion the plethoric twin is at greater risk
B. There is an increased risk of pre-eclampsia
C. There is an increased risk of placenta praevia
D. Dizygotic twins are at greater risk of complications than monozygotic twins
E. Monozygotic twins are always monochorionic

Exam 5: Answers

QUESTION 1

A. FALSE   B. FALSE   C. FALSE   D. FALSE   E. FALSE

An ostium primum ASD results from failure of development of the septum primum, and there is usually also a cleft in the anterior leaflet of the mitral valve. Ostium secundum defects are the most common type of ASD, and these are seen in Holt-Oram syndrome. Ostium primum defects are associated with Down syndrome and Ellis-van-Creveld syndrome.

The defect may be asymptomatic, but can result in heart failure and recurrent pneumonia.

There is a pan-systolic mitral regurgitation murmur, and there is fixed wide splitting of the 2nd heart sound. These defects, unlike many VSDs, require surgical repair.

QUESTION 2

A. TRUE   B. TRUE   C. FALSE   D. TRUE   E. FALSE

Wolf-Parkinson-White (WPW) syndrome is a congenital condition resulting from an abnormal connection between the atria and the ventricles.

The ECG has a short PR interval, wide QRS complexes and a delta wave. There are two types: (a) and (b). Type a is the commonest, and is activation of the left ventricle via the accessory pathway. Type b is activation of the right ventricle via the accessory pathway and occurs with Ebstein's anomaly.

Intermittent episodes of supraventricular tachycardia occur, and there is a risk of VT.

Presentation may be with hydrops foetalis or intra-uterine death if there is in-utero tachycardia.

Flecanide can be used to stop the tachycardia and to reduce the risk of recurrence of tachycardia.

QUESTION 3

A. FALSE   B. FALSE   C. FALSE   D. FALSE   E. TRUE

Tetralogy of Fallot is the most common congenital cyanotic heart condition. It may present with cyanosis in the first few days of life, though this is rare. Usually it presents as a murmur detected in the first few months of life or as hypercyanotic spells in late infancy.

A hot bath will increase cyanosis, as the vasodilation results in a decrease in peripheral vascular resistance, and so the flow through the pulmonary artery decreases, and cyanosis increases. During a cyanotic spell the decrease (not increase) in flow through the pulmonary artery results in the murmur becoming softer or inaudible.

There is a right sided aortic arch in about 30% of cases.

Tetralogy of Fallot is associated with DiGeorge syndrome, and with Down's syndrome, CHARGE syndrome and VACTERL syndrome.

QUESTION 4

A. FALSE   B. TRUE   C. FALSE   D. FALSE   E. TRUE

Infective endocarditis is seen particularly with congenital heart disease, and on previously damaged and prosthetic valves.

It is very uncommon in atrial septal defects, and is seen with high flow defects.

Mycotic aneurysms can occur in both central and peripheral arteries, including cerebral arteries.

Osler's nodes and splinter haemorrhages are both seen uncommonly.

Staphylococcus aureus causes about half of the acute cases. *Streptococcus viridans* causes about half of the cases of subacute bacterial endocarditis.

QUESTION 5

A. FALSE   B. FALSE   C. FALSE   D. TRUE   E. FALSE

Lymphocytic interstitial pneumonia (LIP) is a disease of unknown aetiology. It is seen most commonly in children who have vertically acquired HIV infection. The chest X-ray findings are of a diffuse infiltration and sometimes a perihilar lymphadenopathy also. There may be associated hepatosplenomegaly, generalised lymphadenopathy or pancreatitis. Steroid therapy is only necessary if symptomatic to reduce oxygen requirement and increase exercise tolerance.

QUESTION 6

A. FALSE   B. TRUE   C. FALSE   D. FALSE   E. TRUE

In cystic fibrosis, the underlying defect is in a chloride channel blocker, cystic fibrosis transmembrane regulator (CFTR). The chromosome defect is loss of phenylalanine at position 508 on chromosome 7 in around 80% of cases. The immune reactive trypsin (IRT), used in diagnosis of those under 3 months can be checked on the Guthrie card.

The sweat sodium concentration is the definitive test and this is diagnostic if on two tests the sodium is above 60 mmol/l. False positive sweat tests are seen in ectodermal dysplasia.

QUESTION 7

A. FALSE   B. FALSE   C. FALSE   D. FALSE   E. FALSE

Infants have softer, more compliant ribs, resulting in recession more easily, therefore recession in an older child is more significant.

About 85% of cardiac arrests in children are due to respiratory failure.

The loudness of a wheeze is dependant on both airway diameter and flow. A softening of wheeze may indicate a tiring child (with reduced airway flow).

Basic resuscitation in respiratory failure should be done prior to detailed examination.

Oxygen delivery is variable when given via nasal cannulae.

QUESTION 8

A. TRUE   B. TRUE   C. TRUE   D. FALSE   E. TRUE

IDDM and thyroiditis are endocrine associations but Addison's disease is not recognised as such, although there is a predominance of autoimmune diseases.

Ref: Walker-Smith J. Chapter 27. *Pediatric Gastrointestinal Disease*. Ed Walker et al. Mosby. St Louis. 1996.

QUESTION 9

A. FALSE   B. FALSE   C. FALSE   D. TRUE   E. TRUE

Polygenic inheritance, male > female. Increase in sympathetic activity is due to absence of parasympathetic ganglions in the plexi of Auerbach and Meissner.

QUESTION 10

A. TRUE   B. FALSE   C. FALSE   D. FALSE   E. TRUE

Eye complications occur equally. Sclerosing cholangitis, chronic active hepatitis, cirrhosis, and pericholangitis are all commoner in UC.

Ref: Leichtner A, Jackson W, Grand D. Chapter 27. In: *Pediatric Gastrointestinal Disease*. Ed Walker A et al. St Louis. 1996.

QUESTION 11

A. FALSE   B. FALSE   C. TRUE   D. TRUE   E. FALSE

T_3 is more often low with an apparently normal T_4. Diarrhoea may occur with laxative abuse but constipation is commoner with inherent hypomotility of the gut.

QUESTION 12

A. TRUE   B. TRUE   C. TRUE   D. FALSE   E. FALSE

Haemolytic uraemic syndrome may be triggered by *E. coli* 0157. Factor V Leiden deficiency is present in up to 10% of the Caucasian population and results in a pro-coagulation tendency, which in turn may lead to renal vein thrombosis and haematuria.

QUESTION 13

A. TRUE   B. TRUE   C. TRUE   D. TRUE   E. FALSE

IgA is raised in over 50%. It is a vasculitic phenomenon and this is the cause of the rash, rather than any abnormality of coagulation or platelet function which may lead to a prolonged clotting or bleeding time. Death from massive pulmonary haemorrhage is reported although rare. Opinion on the use of steroids in children with abdominal pain is still divided, as it was felt that they may mask the pain associated with intussusception.

QUESTION 14

A. FALSE   B. FALSE   C. TRUE   D. TRUE   E. TRUE

Cystinosis is associated with Fanconi's syndrome. Do not get **Fanconi's anaemia** confused with **Fanconi's syndrome**.

QUESTION 15

A. FALSE   B. FALSE   C. TRUE   D. FALSE   E. FALSE

Penicillamine causes membranous GN. Most cases of minimal change GN are idiopathic. Initial treatment is prednisolone 60 mg/m^2/day until no proteinuria then alternate days for 4 weeks, but if no response then a renal biopsy is advocated. Abdominal pain is a medical emergency and may indicate hypovolaemia requiring urgent correction, or major vein thrombosis, or primary or pneumococcal peritonitis.

QUESTION 16

A. TRUE   B. FALSE   C. TRUE   D. TRUE   E. FALSE

If children with Alagille's syndrome, usually inherited as an autosomal dominant condition, and also called arteriohepatic dysplasia, require liver transplantation it is due to uncontrollable itching and poor quality of life rather than liver failure which is not common. Zellweger's syndrome (cerebrohepatorenal syndrome) is an example of a peroxisomal disorder but this group does not include Alagille's syndrome. Features of Alagille's include progressive intrahepatic bile duct paucity; intense pruritus; typical facies with hypertelorism, deep set eyes, long nose, broad forehead and small mandible; posterior embryotoxon of the eyes; peripheral pulmonary stenosis and Fallot's tetralogy; tubulointerstitial nephropathy; butterfly vertebrae; tuberous xanthomas and raised serum cholesterol; and it occurs at an incidence of 1 in 100 000 live births. Gene mapping is now possible with a gene defect localised to chromosome 20p (gene termed JAG1) coding for a ligand of Notch 1, which is one of a member of 4 transmembrane proteins.

Ref: Roberts E. Chapter 2. In: *Diseases of the liver and biliary system in childhood*. Ed Kelly D. Blackwell Science. Oxford 1999.

QUESTION 17

A. TRUE   B. FALSE   C. TRUE   D. TRUE   E. FALSE

Normal portal pressure is only 7 mmHg. Caput medusae results in blood flow away from the umbilicus. Perivertebral and perispinal collaterals may occur and *in extremis* may cause signs of spinal compression. Factor V Leiden deficiency occurs in up to 10-15% of the Caucasian population and may result in hypercoagulation and hepatic or portal vein thromboses. As younger children rely, in part, on an increase in their heart rate to counter hypovolaemia secondary to potential haemorrhage from varices, β-blockers are not recommended to decrease portal pressure as this protective mechanism may therefore be compromised.

Ref: Shepherd R. Chapter 11. In: *Diseases of the liver and biliary system in childhood*. Ed Kelly D. Blackwell Science. Oxford 1999.

QUESTION 18

A. TRUE   B. TRUE   C. TRUE   D. TRUE   E. TRUE

A drop in AST/ALT (SGOT/SGPT) can reflect massive hepatocellular necrosis and little residual viable liver tissue. A mitochondrial cytopathy uncovered by sodium valproate is usually responsible for fulminant liver failure in this instance and therefore multisystem involvement including neurological precludes survival even with liver transplant in nearly all cases. Metabolic acidosis may occur, but respiratory alkalosis also occurs in stage II-III encephalopathy. Coagulation is a good indicator of liver function and should not be artificially supported unless necessary. Vitamin K and the liver's response to it may yield useful information.

Ref: N Shah and M Thomson. Liver. In: *Paediatric Intensive Care*. 1999.

QUESTION 19

A. TRUE   B. TRUE   C. TRUE   D. FALSE   E. TRUE

Plasma cholesterol reflects liver synthetic function, like serum albumin and coagulation state, and if it is low this reflects worsening liver function and poorer prognosis. Neurodevelopmental delay, and other subtle symptoms such as school problems or lethargy can reflect chronic hepatic encephalopathy. Spontaneous bacterial peritonitis should always be suspected in children with ascites, abdominal pain and fever. Paracentesis reveals cloudy fluid with a neutrophil count of > 250/ml. *Klebsiella*, *E. coli* or *Strep. pneumoniae* predominate.

Ref: Shepherd R. Chapter 11. In: *Diseases of the liver and biliary system in childhood*. Ed Kelly D. Blackwell Science. Oxford 1999.

QUESTION 20

A. TRUE   B. TRUE   C. TRUE   D. TRUE   E. TRUE

All the above are seen in intravascular haemolyisis, which is the destruction of red cells within the circulation. The particular features of intravascular haemolysis are:

- Haemoglobinaemia
- Haemoglobinuria
- Haemosiderinuria
- Methaemoglobinaemia
- Red cell fragments

QUESTION 21

A. TRUE   B. FALSE   C. TRUE   D. TRUE   E. TRUE

Homozygous sickle cell disease does not usually present in infancy. Features include painful crises, haemolytic crises, acute sequestration and aplastic crises. Painful crises (vascular-occlusive) occur in the bones (most commonly). The other organs may also be involved including the kidney, liver, spleen, heart, brain and chest. Painful swollen fingers (dactylitis) may be seen, with bony infarcts resulting in different length fingers. Other features include pigment gallstones, leg ulcers, salmonella osteomyelitis and proliferative retinopathy.

QUESTION 22

A. TRUE   B. TRUE   C. TRUE   D. TRUE   E. FALSE

The bleeding time measures platelet plug formation in vivo. A prolonged bleeding time is seen in thombocytopaenia and in platelet function disorders. These include:

Bernard-Soulier syndrome (platelet adhesion defect, few large platelets)

Glanzmann's disease (Failure of platelet aggregation due to a deficiency of membrane glycoproteins IIb and IIIa.)

Hermansky-Pudlak syndrome (platelet function disorder and albinism)

von Willebrand's disease (platelet adhesion abnormalities present)

The bleeding time is normal in Haemophilia A and B.

QUESTION 23

A. FALSE   B. TRUE   C. TRUE   D. TRUE   E. TRUE

The causes of thrombocytopaenia in the neonatal period are many. They may be due to an increased consumption of platelets or decreased production.

Bernard-Soulier syndrome is a disorder of platelet function not numbers. Congenital infections can result in neonatal thrombocytopaenia, and the infant may have a purpuric rash. Neonatal leukaemia is a rare condition.

Renal vein thrombosis and giant haemangiomas result in platelet fall due to a consumptive coagulopathy.

QUESTION 24

A. FALSE   B. FALSE   C. TRUE   D. FALSE   E. FALSE

Osteosarcoma is a spindle cell neoplasm (Ewing's tumour is a small cell tumour). It occurs mainly in the metaphyses of the long bones, particularly the proximal femur and the distal tibia. It is associated with retinoblastoma and osteogenesis imperfecta. It is more common than Ewing's tumour. The X-ray findings are sclerotic lesions and skip lesions (lytic lesions are seen in Ewing's tumour).

QUESTION 25

A. TRUE   B. TRUE   C. FALSE   D. TRUE   E. FALSE

Acute myeloid leukaemia (AML) has many subtypes classified by the French-American-British (FAB) system. Gum hypertrophy is seen particularly in M4 and M5 types and DIC in M3 type. The M3 type has a good prognosis and may be treated with retinoic acid as initial therapy. Fanconi anaemia is associated with AML, as is trisomy 21 and Bloom syndrome. Auer rods are not always seen, depending on the type of ALL.

QUESTION 26

A. TRUE   B. FALSE   C. TRUE   D. TRUE   E. FALSE

Bruton's X-linked agammaglobulinaemia is an X-linked recessive disorder of humoral immunity. The gene defect is a mutation in the btk gene which is on the X chromosome and results in an absence of tyrosine kinase. There is defective transformation of pre-B cells to B cells. The disease presents with recurrent bacterial infections and there may be unusual enteroviral infections (e.g. chronic encephalomyelitis). Pneumocystis carinii infection is seen in T cell immunodeficiency. Regular immunoglobulin infusions (3-4 weekly) are necessary throughout life.

QUESTION 27

A. FALSE   B. FALSE   C. TRUE   D. FALSE   E. TRUE

Job's syndrome (also known as Hyper IgE syndrome), is a syndrome of very high levels of IgE, eczema and recurrent staphylococcal abscesses in the skin, joints and lungs. Small platelets are seen in Wiskott-Aldrich syndrome. The mutations in Jak 3 result in autosomal recessive T-, B+ SCID.

QUESTION 28

A. TRUE   B. FALSE   C. TRUE   D. FALSE   E. FALSE

The haemophilus influenza b (Hib) vaccine is composed of the polysaccharide coat and a protein to make it antigenic. It provides protection to the encapsulated organism haemophilus influenza. This protects from acute epiglottitis and meningitis. It is not a live vaccine. It is not effective in the neonate because maternal Hib antibodies interfere with its effect.

QUESTION 29

A. FALSE   B. TRUE   C. FALSE   D. TRUE   E. TRUE

Mumps virus is one of the paramyxoviruses which are RNA viruses. It is a very common cause of viral meningitis.

It usually involves the parotid gland (60%) or both the parotid and submandibular. It is rare to only involve the submandibular gland. It is a cause of both pancreatitis and myocarditis.

QUESTION 30

A. FALSE   B. TRUE   C. FALSE   D. FALSE   E. FALSE

Plasmodium vivax and *P. ovale* affect the young red blood cells. *P. malariae* affects the old red blood cells. *Plasmodium falciparum* does not have a latent phase in the liver unlike *P. vivax* and *P. ovale*. Schizont rupture releases merozoites. Primaquine is not needed for liver eradication in *P. malariae* infection as there is no latent phase in the liver.

QUESTION 31

A. FALSE   B. TRUE   C. FALSE   D. TRUE   E. FALSE

Leprosy is caused by *Mycobacterium leprae*. It is very slow growing and the incubation period is 3-5 years.

The lepromin test is a measure of host resistance to disease, and is negative in Lepromatous leprosy where the host cell-mediated immunity is poor. The clinical features of the disease are dependent on the immune status of the host, and tuberculoid leprosy is seen in people with a good immune response.

QUESTION 32

A. FALSE   B. TRUE   C. FALSE   D. FALSE   E. FALSE

CSF glucose:plasma ratio is low in bacterial meningitis. Subdural effusions occur in 10-15% of cases of bacterial meningitis.

Kernig sign is often negative in children, especially young infants.

Up to a fifth of infants will present with seizures, and a further fifth will have seizures later on.

Rifampicin is given to contatcs of *N. meningitidis* and *H. influenzae* meningitis, but not *S.pneumoniae*.

QUESTION 33

A. FALSE   B. FALSE   C. TRUE   D. TRUE   E. TRUE

Galactosaemia has an incidence of 1 in 60 000. The enzyme deficiency is of galactose-1-phosphate uridyl transferase (GAL-1-PUT). This results in an inability to metabolise galactose (and thus also lactose, which is made of glucose + galactose).

Clinical features include presentation as a neonate with vomiting, hypoglycaemia, feeding difficulties, neurological features and liver disorder. Diagnosis is by enzyme assay in RBCs. Non-glucose reducing substances are seen in the urine when milk fed (i.e. Clinitest positive, Clinistix negative). The Guthrie tests for galactosaemia.

Management involves a lactose and galactose free diet. Speech-language problems and ovarian failure though, are almost inevitable even with therapy.

QUESTION 34

A. TRUE   B. TRUE   C. TRUE   D. TRUE   E. TRUE

The mitochondrial disorders may indeed present at any age and by any mode of inheritance. They are usually autosomal recessive. They include MERRF, Pearson's syndrome, MELAS (mitochondrial myopathy, encephalopathy, lactic acidosis and stroke-like episodes) syndrome and Leigh's syndrome.

Diagnosis is suggested by an elevated free-floating blood lactate in the absence of sepsis, hypoxia, poor tissue perfusion or other metabolic disorder which causes high lactate. Diagnosis is confirmed by enzyme analysis.

Features are many and variable, and they include retinitis pigmentosa.

QUESTION 35

A. FALSE   B. TRUE   C. FALSE   D. TRUE   E. FALSE

X-linked adrenoleucodystrophy is a peroxisomal disorder of very long chain fatty acid (VLCFA) oxidation. It results in progressive adrenal cortex and neuronal white matter degeneration, and the phenotype is variable. It may present with Addison's disease, or it may present with neurological features (behaviour disturbance, developmental regression, ataxia, seizures, spasticity).

Diagnostic investigations include VLCFAs, adrenal cortical function tests, MRI brain scan and neuropsychiatric assessment.

Management is supportive with adrenal steroid replacement, anticonvulsants, NG or gastrostomy feeding. Supplementation with monounsaturated amino acids (Lorenzo's oil) may be beneficial but is not curative.

QUESTION 36

A. TRUE   B. FALSE   C. FALSE   D. TRUE   E. FALSE

Congenital hypothyroidism occurs with an incidence of around 1 in 4 000. It is most commonly due to thyroid dysgenesis with ectopic thyroid tissue. Dyshormonogenesis accounts for only about 10% of cases. Maternal hyperthyroidism may result in congenital hypothyroidism through antibodies crossing the placenta, or from the antithyroid drugs. Significant intellectual impairment is avoidable if hormone therapy is instituted early.

QUESTION 37

A. TRUE   B. FALSE   C. TRUE   D. TRUE   E. TRUE

The causes of diabetes insipidus may be separated into intracranial causes and nephrogenic causes. Craniopharyngioma and neonatal listeriosis are causes of intracranial diabetes insipidus. DIDMOAD syndrome stands for diabetes insipidus, diabetes mellitus, optic atrophy and deafness. Demeclocycline can cause nephrogenic diabetes insipidus. Carbamazepine is used in the treatment of nephrogenic diabetes insipidus.

QUESTION 38

A. FALSE   B. FALSE   C. TRUE   D. TRUE   E. FALSE

Craniopharyngioma is one of the most common supratentorial tumours in childhood (not infratentorial). It may present with the hormonal effects of hypopituitarism, including growth failure, polyuria (due to diabetes insipidus), hypothyroidism and adrenocortical insufficiency. It arises from a remnant of the connection between the Rathke's pouch and the oral cavity. In most cases there is calcification on the skull X-ray.

QUESTION 39

A. FALSE   B. FALSE   C. FALSE   D. FALSE   E. FALSE

In familial hypophosphataemic rickets (also known as vitamin D-resistant rickets), there is defective proximal renal tubular reabsorption of phosphate, and a reduced synthesis of 1,25-hydroxycholecalciferol. Plasma levels of PTH are normal, and calcium is normal or low. Plasma phosphate levels are low. The inheritance is X-linked dominant.

QUESTION 40

A. TRUE   B. FALSE   C. FALSE   D. FALSE   E. FALSE

Children with autism demonstrate repetitive behaviour, have poor eye contact with others, and have a very poor emotional bond with both their mother and other people. The EEG is usually normal. They have normal motor development, but their speech is delayed with difficulty understanding language.

QUESTION 41

A. FALSE   B. TRUE   C. TRUE   D. FALSE   E. FALSE

Febrile convulsions occur in around 2-5% of children and are more common in males. They occur between 6 months and 6 years. They are associated with an increased risk of later development of epilepsy, particularly if atypical and there is a family history of epilepsy. There is a positive family history of febrile convulsions in around 30% of cases.

QUESTION 42

A. FALSE   B. TRUE   C. TRUE   D. FALSE   E. TRUE

Late Infantile Batten's Disease (Ceroid Lipofuscinosis) is an autosomal recessive condition. The features are normal early development then developmental regression from around 2-5 years. There is a chronic ataxia and retinitis pigmentosa can occur. Typical neurological features are seen on histology of rectal biopsy.

QUESTION   43

A. TRUE   B. FALSE   C. TRUE   D. TRUE   E. TRUE

Raised intracranial pressure may develop insidiously or rapidly, and drowsiness is a feature of a rapidly rising pressure. Convulsions are an unusual presentation in children. The headache is worse on lying down and in the mornings. There may be a sixth nerve palsy (a false localising sign). Signs take longer to develop in young children as the cranial sutures can widen.

QUESTION   44

A. FALSE   B. TRUE   C. TRUE   D. FALSE   E. FALSE

Slipped upper femoral epiphysis is seen most commonly in adolescents. It is associated with hypothyroidism and other pituitary dysfunction. It may present with referred pain from the knee. The hip X-ray shows widening of the growth plate as the head 'slips' off the neck.

Examination reveals decreased internal rotation of the hip, and the hip is chronically externally rotated.

QUESTION   45

A. FALSE   B. TRUE   C. TRUE   D. FALSE   E. FALSE

Chloroquine may be given in G6PD deficiency though haemolysis can occur in some forms of the disease; dapsone and sulphur containing drugs should be avoided. Proguanil acts by inhibiting folate production, and the parasital cells cannot utilise tetrahydrofolate from external sources unlike mammalian cells. Pyrimethamine resistance is high and it is no longer recommended as prophylaxis for travellers. Long term chloroquine is associated with corneal opacities and retinal damage.

QUESTION   46

A. TRUE   B. TRUE   C. TRUE   D. TRUE   E. FALSE

Doxorubicin is a naturally occurring anthracycline and derived from streptomyces. It is effective against solid tumours and is part of the regime of many solid tumours. It induces free radical formation which cardiac cells specifically cannot deal with; the clinical effects though are variable. Doxorubicin binds to DNA and alters the DNA helix shape, thus inhibiting DNA polymerase. There is a risk of severe infection with disseminated zoster in patients with a history of shingles.

QUESTION   47

A. TRUE   B. TRUE   C. TRUE   D. TRUE   E. TRUE

All of these are liver enzyme inducers. Brussel sprouts and barbecued meat both act as liver enzyme inducers. Heavy smoking and drinking may account for a failure to respond to a normal drug dose.

QUESTION   48

A. TRUE   B. FALSE   C. TRUE   D. TRUE   E. TRUE

Hypoventilation is a late feature of salicylate poisoning, and together with coma indicates severe poisoning. The acid-base disturbances are complex and both acidosis and alkalosis may occur. Salicylates have a direct stimulant effect on the respiratory centre resulting in hyperventilation and a respiratory alkalosis seen early on, though this stage may not be apparent in young infants.

QUESTION   49

A. TRUE   B. TRUE   C. FALSE   D. TRUE   E. TRUE

Mollusca contagiosa is a common infection among school children caused by a pox virus. It presents as pearly papules with a central umbilicus. Spontaneous resolution usually occurs within 6-9 months, though the lesions can last for years. Disseminated infection may be seen in children with atopic eczema and in the immunosuppressed. No treatment is usually given as this can result in scarring, however, cryotherapy is a treatment option if necessary.

QUESTION   50

A. TRUE   B. FALSE   C. TRUE   D. TRUE   E. FALSE

Reiter's syndrome is an acute reactive arthritis. It follows gastrointestinal infection (including *Campylobacter, Shigella, Yersinia, Salmonella*) or venereal infection (chlamydia or NSU).

It has a high male preponderance, and is associated with HLA-B27 (80%).

Features include a lower limb arthritis, which may become chronic, occular inflammation and a sterile urethritis. Other features are keratoderma blenorrhagica, plantar fasciitis, entheseopathy, nail dystrophy and mouth ulceration.

Treatment is with antibiotics, physiotherapy and NSAIDS.

QUESTION   51

A. TRUE   B. FALSE   C. FALSE   D. FALSE   E. FALSE

Kawasaki disease is an infantile polyarteritis. The diagnostic criteria are a fever of > 38.5°C for > 5 days together with 4 of the following features:

- Bilateral non-purulent conjunctivitis
- Oral mucosal changes
- Cervical lymphadenopathy with one node > 1.5 cm
- Involvement of hands and feet with erythema, swelling or peeling of the palms and soles
- Rash (polymorphous)

The child is usually extremely irritable, with cough or coryzal symptoms, and may have watery diarrhoea.

Cardiac complications are a significant cause of morbidity. Coronary artery aneurysms occur in up to 20% of children who are not treated.

A thrombocythaemia is seen in the second and third weeks, and a high WCC and anaemia may be seen.

Management is with high dose intravenous immunoglobulin over 12 hours, which should be given within 10 days of disease onset. Aspirin is given for 6 weeks or until the coronary aneurysms are gone, which is assessed by echocardiogram at follow-up.

QUESTION   52

A. FALSE   B. TRUE   C. FALSE   D. TRUE   E. TRUE

Syndromes involoving absent radii include:

- Holt-Oram syndrome
- Fanconi anaemia
- VATER syndrome

- TAR syndrome
- Absent thumbs

QUESTION 53

A. TRUE   B. TRUE   C. TRUE   D. TRUE   E. TRUE

Noonan syndrome is inherited in an autosomal dominant fashion, though most cases are sporadic. The appearance may be similar to Turner's syndrome and features include:

- Mental retardation (in 25%)
- Ptosis
- Epicanthic folds
- Hypertelorism
- Down-slanting palpebral fissures
- Cardiac defects: these include valvular pulmonary stenosis, PDA, VSD and peripheral pulmonary stenosis

QUESTION 54

A. FALSE   B. FALSE   C. FALSE   D. FALSE   E. TRUE

The lung bud is an outgrowth from the foregut and derived from endodermal tissue. The respiratory bronchioles develop from about 17 weeks gestation and surfactant production can be detected by about 23 weeks gestation. The type II pneumocytes produce surfactant.

QUESTION 55

A. TRUE   B. TRUE   C. FALSE   D. TRUE   E. TRUE

Multifactorial inheritance involves both genetic and environmental factors. Many diseases have multifactorial inheritance including cleft lip and palate, pyloric stenosis, neural tube defects, club foot and congenital hip dislocation. Empirical recurrence risks are based on studies of large collections of families. The risk increases if more family members are affected, if the disease has more severe expression and if the affected case is a member of the less commonly affected sex.

QUESTION 56

A. FALSE   B. FALSE   C. TRUE   D. FALSE   E. FALSE

A single blind trial is one in which either the patient or the assessor, but not both, does not know which group the patient has been assigned to.

The Chi-squared test is carried out using numerical data only and not percentages.

Randomisation will help eliminate selection bias because it ensures all patients should have an equal chance of being assigned to each group.

The median is the value which divides the range of values into two equal parts.

The incidence of a disorder is the number of new cases occurring over a set period of time.

QUESTION 57

A. FALSE   B. FALSE   C. TRUE   D. FALSE   E. FALSE

Human breast milk contains more carbohydrate, more iron, less protein than cow's milk, and it has a lower casein to whey ratio.

It is a poor source of vitamin K and is therefore a risk factor for haemorrhagic disease of the newborn.

QUESTION 58

A. TRUE   B. TRUE   C. FALSE   D. TRUE   E. TRUE

Conditions associated with premature closure of the fontanelle include many skeletal disorders, such as achondroplasia, Apert syndrome and osteogenesis imperfecta. Progeria is also associated with delayed closure of the fontanelle. Malnutrition may result in delayed closure. Other conditions associated with delayed closure include Trisomy 13, Trisomy 18 and Trisomy 21.

Hyperthyroidism is associated with premature closure, and hypothyroidism with delayed closure of the fontanelle.

QUESTION 59

A. TRUE   B. TRUE   C. TRUE   D. FALSE   E. FALSE

Neonatal hypocalcaemia is seen in infants of diabetic mothers, and in infants with birth asphyxia. Infants fed on cow's milk formula can develop hypocalcaemia because this milk is very high in phosphate which the neonatal kidney cannot manage to excrete. This results in increased bone deposition of calcium, decreased 1,25-dihydroxyVitamin D levels, and hypocalcaemia.

Hypomagnasaemia and neonatal hypoparathyroidism will result in hypocalcaemia.

QUESTION 60

A. TRUE   B. TRUE   C. TRUE   D. FALSE   E. FALSE

In twin-twin transfusion the larger plethoric twin is the one at greater risk of a number of complications.

There is an increased risk of almost everything in twin pregnancy, including pre-eclampsia and placenta praevia.

Monozygotic twins are at greater risk than dizygotic because if the chorion is shared there are risks of vascular anastomoses with twin-twin transfusion and cord entangling. Monozygotic twins, may, however, be dichorionic.